Things Are Going Great In My Absence

How To Let Go And Let The Divine

Do The Heavy Lifting

Lola Jones

www.DivineOpenings.com
admin@lolajones.com

www.DivineOpenings.de
support@DivineOpeningsGermany.com

This book is not intended to replace your own inner guidance,
nor to provide or replace medical or other professional advice.

Published by Lola Jones.
Printed in the United States of America.

ISBN: 978-1-7323994-0-2

Acknowledgments and Appreciation

While most of the content of this book was given from within and was more profound and effective than anything I'd ever learned from others, parts of it were catalyzed by great teachers and powerful initiations from this lifetime and others. It would be impossible to name all the generous, wise, and wonderful people who helped shape this life and assisted my spiritual expansion before and since Divine Openings. Those who've expanded my heart and mind are many, including the many readers of this book, our worldwide community, and the attendees of our live retreats who expand this leading edge.

I feel tremendous appreciation for Donna Wetterstrand of Canada, Melinda Gates of Texas, Emily Colwell of North Carolina, and Angelika Lukoschek of Germany, Divine Openings Mentors who train our Certified Guides and contribute so much to Divine Openings. Appreciation to all who have shared Divine Openings so generously all over the world.

Endless love and appreciation to Scott Sanderson, who told me when we met, "I will open *you* up like you open other people up." He did indeed.

We create each other on this journey.
You ask and the teacher appears.

Appreciation to all the many thousands of you who grace my life.

I love you.

IMPORTANT NOTE:

To insure the quality and purity of Divine Openings,

Lola Jones is the only person who can certify others to give Divine Openings.

Things Are Going Great In My Absence:
How To Let Go And Let The Divine Do The Heavy Lifting

By Lola Jones

A dramatic awakening is happening on the planet right now. Human consciousness is expanding exponentially. Those of us out on the leading edge are experiencing a rapid expansion of consciousness—right now. We invite you to join us on a safe and nurturing yet exciting path to freedom and happiness.

Whatever you want next in your life, this book will help you achieve it with more ease, Grace, and flow. You get help on two levels: the Grace piece and the conscious mind piece. The Grace piece is most powerful by far. You receive Divine Grace, which by definition is a gift you cannot earn, but is freely given. It lifts you higher than you could humanly lift yourself. Much of the process is effortless for you when you let Grace do at least 90% of the work. Your small 10% (the conscious mind piece) is to learn how to soften, let it in, and get out of the way. We show you precisely how. You receive tools you can use to consciously make more powerful, effective choices.

Receive a series of initiations to enlightenment, or a deepening of your enlightenment, as you read this book, gaze at the illustrations in it, and feel the Divine Presence in it—the Divine Presence that is in you. You will want everyone you know and care about to get this book, so they can share this bountiful experience with you and join you in this wondrous new world.

Once the Divine Presence in you is awake and walking this planet as *You*, once you are in the flow of life that supplies all wants and needs, creating the life you want is easy, fun, joyful, and exciting. Suffering, conflict, and struggle cease. Synchronicities become commonplace as you come together with people, resources, and events for mutual benefit and sharing of joy.

Once seeking is over and true living begins, you live in confidence, relish the moment, and create what you want. The "power of now" is a tangible reality rather than a wishful concept or something to work toward. The past and the future have no hold on you, and loss, worry, and scarcity can no longer be found.

You are "unsinkable" when you live as your Large Self, and truly feel the power of who you are. Crime, government, heartbreak, money issues—nothing has power over you in this new paradigm. People around you literally transform because of who you are, and you never feel powerless to make a difference again, yet you know when to let go.

Begin right now to enjoy a more vital, personal relationship with your Creator, who is eager and waiting to co-create more closely with you to fulfill all of your heart's desires.

Lola Jones spent twenty-one delicious days in solitary, silent retreat in early 2006, communing only with the Presence Within, and a lifetimes-old gift was reactivated within her. She now invokes a potent form of Grace that activates awakening or deepens enlightenment. It changes people's lives dramatically. She can light people up by touching them, activate the Energy/Light/Intelligence by intention in group settings, convey it by voice on the phone or webinar at any distance—and people feel its effects powerfully through this book. You'll experience it directly as you gaze at the art, read the words, and sit in the powerful vortex this book creates.

Lola's "job" to get out of the way and let The Divine do the heavy lifting. She is often almost "absent" from the process as she helps others, even as she enjoys the blissful sensations of it. She also found that as The Divine in her woke up and she lived more fully as her Large Self, her own practical daily life continued to get easier and easier. Her Larger Self increasingly runs her life as her small self takes a back seat and relaxes, hence the title: *Things Are Going Great In My Absence.*

In reading this chronicle of Lola's own awakening, and experiencing the simple activities, the Divine Intelligence in you gradually wakes up or expands. You learn how to receive it, what to expect in the process, how to get out of the way, allow it to be easier, and sustain it.

IMPORTANT

On your first reading, this book is best read in order,
slowly, from front to back. This is potent, powerful material, and
you need to absorb the instructions before receiving the first Divine Opening,
and to understand the unfolding that follows. "Rushing" reduces
your results dramatically in this reading, and in Life. It's not about gaining knowledge.

Experience it, feel it, live it, bit by bit—deeply.

As this evolutionary energy evolves and accelerates, it changes and upgrades rapidly. To receive updates, enlightening gifts, articles, news, events, and inspiration simply join the email list at DivineOpenings.com/aweber.

This book is the foundation of Divine Openings. If you should wish to access voluminous additional material, support, multi-media, audios, and videos, refer to DivineOpenings.com or DivineOpenings.de.

Ready? You are about to enter a new reality.

Table Of Contents

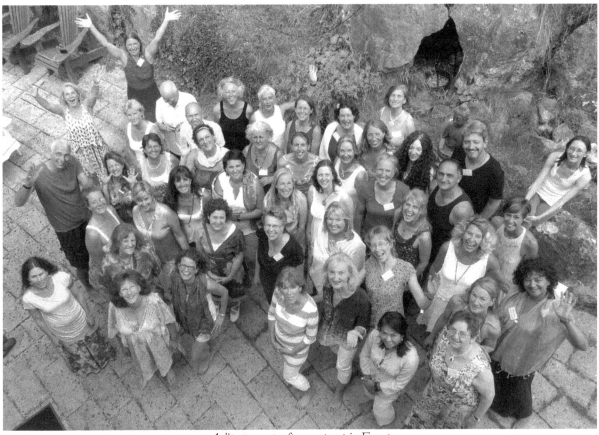

A lit-up group after a retreat in Europe.

Things Are Going Great in My Absence:
How To Let Go And Let The Divine Do The Heavy Lifting

How and Why I Wrote This Book

THIS BOOK FLOWED out of me naturally and effortlessly. I didn't will the book to happen; it willed me to write it and I could not stop. That's how everything has gone this past twelve years. My body does what it wants to. It paints or writes when it wants to, or not. Sometimes I write all day and forget to eat. My old concepts of ambition and motivation don't make much sense to me anymore. Things that used to seem important are not. Life lives *through* me. I mostly go along for the ride, watching the beautiful scenery go by, and enjoying the wonderful adventures on the way. It's the best ride of my life.

As more of the Divine Intelligence in you wakes up and takes over, as outer changes unfold and the old reality unravels, as emotions arise and move on, this book helps your mind understand what's going on. You participated in the creation of this book—you asked for it in your heart. The Divine Openings process doesn't require your mind's understanding, but your unfolding is accelerated when the mind *cooperates* rather than *resists*. This book retrains, guides, and soothes your mind during this time of change. Until your inner knowing has flowered more completely, it helps to have some guidance navigating the changes and integrating it into your daily life. Let in the help and opening, but please, always trust your own guidance and intuition over anyone's, including mine.

This book embodies my experience successfully helping many thousands of people in more than 150 countries access their own truths and awaken to their own oneness with The Divine Intelligence within. It's unlike any book you've ever read—far beyond just intellectual concepts, it's an *experience* that alters your entire way of living.

The Light Emerges

WHILE GIVING DIVINE OPENINGS at a public event, going from one person to the next, touching each person for about two minutes, five of them reported seeing a brilliant white light through their closed eyelids as I stood in front of them. The normal expectation would be that someone standing in front of you would cause your field of vision to darken. (Try it!) They were seeing my light body. When I am with people, one-to-one or in a group, a powerful vortex opens that activates or deepens their awakening, and they realign more and more with the Pure Life Force that has always been inside of them. They awaken to what's not visible in the physical world. None of this is to say I am special—it is to demonstrate that many of us human beings are quite literally becoming less dense and more purely light. The kinds of experiences you read about here are possible for you, and will eventually happen as you practice Divine Openings, learn to go within for your needs, and don't dilute it.

Jesus and Mary were often depicted with a halo of light around their heads. It was promised we would all one day be as they were, do the things they were able to do, and more. You will experience "miracles," which are actually commonplace when you're in the flow of Life. What has been called "ascension" is the completed transformation of our bodies and minds so we become less dense. We are "en-lightening." Lightening up! Becoming more spacious.

As the light in each of us radiates more brightly, it becomes more visible. We normally think of the function of eyes as receptors of light, because light goes into them. After a person's awakening begins, I notice their eyes lighting up—light is coming *from* their eyes, not just going *into* their eyes. In the first year I created Divine Openings, I formally opened about seven hundred people hands-on, in small groups and retreats. Many thousands have received it through this book. I've noticed it beginning to affect people after merely having dinner with them. If I see that happening, I offer this book so they'll understand the changes taking place, and so they can use their Free Will to reduce resistance to the Grace.

The Energy/Light/Intelligence of Divine Openings continually amps up; and as more and more people "light up," or "en-lighten," the whole collective consciousness of humanity lightens just a bit. People reading this book begin to see their own enlightenment reflected in their families, friends, co-workers, communities as a rapid, spontaneous quickening, a chain reaction of awakening takes place.

The experience of unfolding is the real adventure. Slow down and enjoy every single moment! This is not going to be "work." As you enlighten, you help humanity without doing or teaching anything. Those of us on this frontier break the waves for those who come after. Most won't know you helped them, just as Americans don't know the names of each of the hardy American pioneers who paved the way to the New World for them. The ones who come along in your energetic footprints will benefit from your courage and foresight, and on the Larger level, they are You.

My friend related a story about a fellow karate master and teacher, a man's man who never studied metaphysics and was not on a spiritual path, who had a spontaneous enlightenment experience while he was alone in nature, in the mountains. Love suddenly enveloped him, tears flowed, and a sense of wonder and awe overtook him. He didn't know what was happening. Wondering who he knew that was weird enough to understand this, he confided in my friend, searching for explanations for this strange and unexpected change. The two men talked for two hours. He told of giving his wife flowers for the first time in decades, upon which she inquired, "Okay, who is she?" She thought he must have had an affair! He'd found new love all right, but it was Divine Love.

The karate master's awakening occurred through a mysterious, spontaneous opening. Precious few ever find it through seeking or toiling on some spiritual path. Now Divine Openings gives you the opportunity to receive it by Grace, rather than hoping it happens someday before you die.

That man's state remains transformed, but I often help people who had such enlightenment experiences and could not sustain them until Divine Openings. One Buddhist (not a reader of this book) had a full-blown enlightenment experience that lasted for six months, until an encounter with his mother brought him crashing down!

Things Are Going Great In My Absence gives not only the awakening energy and the enlightenment initiations but the structure and support to maintain it. Our human mind and our outer world certainly don't validate or support it. I know of a few people who were temporarily committed to psychiatric hospitals after spontaneous, unexpected bursts of oneness and enlightenment. As they marveled wide-eyed at the dancing leaves on the trees and the light emanating from everything, no one around them understood what was happening to them—and neither did they. That fear and confusion needn't happen when you undertake the process deliberately, with proper guidance and understanding. You can have a very functional enlightenment.

Once the awakening process begins, the most common early effect we hear is that anxiety disappears, replaced by a deep inexplicable knowing that all is well (the "peace that passes understanding.") The mind may at first want to control, define, or explain away Divine Openings, but as we grow accustomed to operating beyond the limited mind we relax into the Mystery.

Questions are answered most often from within, solutions arise effortlessly, with the occasional message or help coming serendipitously from someone or something outside. Striving stops, and there is a peace with the present moment and the "perfect imperfection" of our humanity.

There is still curiosity and desire (oh, yes, passionate desire) but frantic, lackful seeking ceases. The urge to grow and expand is eternal, but the days of fruitless striving for it are over. Now you can stop working on yourself, healing issues, or needing someone to fix you.

I remind you several times to read *slowly* because people are so conditioned to read books in a mad rush, thinking the faster they can suck up the information, the sooner they can get on to the next book. That leads to shallow, futile, perpetual seeking. Speeding on is an unconscious tactic to avoid deep feeling and actual experience. Slow down.

Even "advanced" people don't get everything the first time through this book. People say each subsequent reading is a next-level experience. That's because your consciousness expands between readings. Divine Openings empties you out rather than filling your head with more intellectual knowledge. You get lighter, freer, and more spacious rather than more full of mind-stuff. When you're tapped into the Flow of Life, you don't need to drag along a lot of luggage on your journey, what you need shows up in the moment.

Divine Openings increases your capacity to tap into direct knowing. Spiritual and metaphysical theory, books, healings, and ancient texts are replaced with personal experience, direct downloads, automatic evolution, and a living, breathing communion with a vast Intelligence.

Then what you choose to do with it and how you choose to live are completely up to you. The choices are limitless. I don't live by any spiritual stereotype, and you don't have to either.

Soon you will experience yourself "lighter."

What Happens with Divine Openings?

HOW DIVINE OPENINGS WORKS is beyond intellectual comprehension. People sometimes tell me they met me in a dream (sometimes I'm on my white horse!) right before they stumbled across my website or book. Our Non-Physical meeting prepared them to recognize me and Divine Openings in the physical. While I'm asleep my Large Self visits people in my light body and helps them. All I usually remember are abstract, geometric, or other-dimensional dreams.

My greatest gift is the ability to get completely out of the way and let the power of Divine Openings use me without any need to understand, define, or dissect it into something small enough to fit in a human brain. Nowhere in this book will you find a scientific rationale for it, because I don't care about that. My playground is the Mystery out beyond science.

Since Divine Openings, my intellectual capacity has expanded dramatically, but it's not where the greatest power resides. Intellectual concepts that can be explained in words pale in comparison to pure energy and *"direct knowing"* from within—which is knowing without knowing *how* I know. That's why this isn't an ordinary book. A Mystery beyond words lights you up, opens you to larger realities, and changes your life (unless you resist really hard—I'm smiling right now.)

Divine Openings opens you up so you can let in the Grace that always is and always was raining down on you. It simply reveals to you what was already there and who you already are. Everything truly real *is invisible and Non-Physical...* love, joy, vibration, The Divine within you. The invisible begins to be perceptible. It's the opposite of the "physical reality worship" most of the world practices. The physical world stops ruling you as you have direct experiences and tangible knowing of the Non-Physical world. You open and "get it" more with each reading of this book.

For years, the very word "God" made me cringe due to all the fanatics, evangelists, and extremists who have used that word to abuse and judge others. Now, I can finally say it again without tensing up. Notice how the word God makes you feel. If there's a negative conditioned response, it will subside. I'll use many other terms for God, but for ease and brevity I use the word God a lot in this book, yet no word can begin to describe the Mystery. In my private life it needs no name or label—I am enfolded in it.

As you develop a closer, more intimate personal relationship with God, it will impact your health, your finances, your love life, your family relationships, and your entire world in a stunningly tangible, practical way because God cares about your ordinary life circumstances. If you assimilate and practice what's in this book—focusing consistently on Divine Openings for a year, and don't dilute it with other stuff, you won't recognize your life at the end of that year.

I've taught for decades, and Divine Openings has opened people up faster and easier than anything before. It has quite effortlessly removed obstacles and issues that neither the student nor I could perceive. You will find masses and layers of psychological conditioning lifting, and you may never know why or how. You'll just find yourself feeling lighter, freer and happier. Your life blooms, and Divine Intelligence begins to express as you, revealing your unique genius.

Before Divine Openings, in addition to teaching and helping others in personal and corporate settings, I had done *way* too many years getting "cleared" and "healed." The more I cleared, the more showed up to clear. It was never-ending! Finally I said, "Enough! I want a path of joy, not work!" Then Divine Openings emerged, and massive change took place in my life without working on it at all. I felt more powerful and at peace than ever before. I also got healthier, more successful, confident, and happy. No more processing, analyzing, or figuring it all out.

Now it's so obvious looking back that "working on myself" had focused on what was wrong, and so created more issues than it relieved. When I let go and let The Divine do the heavy lifting, my life as a powerful creator began. I'm not saying Divine Openings is the only way—there is no one way for all. *I am saying it works.* If I found a better way, I'd switch instantly—but I have no reason to seek—my unfolding is now natural, easy, happy, and rapid.

When you feel and know who you *really are* deep within, not just in your head—a physical expression of a vast Non-Physical life force—you discover *all* of your old "issues" and limits were *illusory*. Slashing away at illusions for the rest of your life begins to seem rather silly and unnecessary.

There've been many surprises. I had thought of myself more as a teacher, counselor, and enlightener, so I was at first quite surprised by the physical healings that occurred spontaneously during some of the Divine Openings. Although people didn't tell me about their physical problem, The

Presence knew!

Here are just a few comments from people who have received Divine Openings.
Please don't expect the same experience as anyone else. Your unique experience is designed for you.
I adore my own deep, subtle experiences. I also revel in hearing yours!

In their own words:

I have taken two of Lola's seminars, seven years ago, and recently. Both seminars made a HUGE difference in my life. I can honestly say that there were amazing shifts in my life after each course. —M.Z. was on Oprah

I wanted more of God's spirit . . . so now here's more I can receive easier by Grace through Divine Openings, untainted by religious doctrine. Blessings, —Bev McCaw

I am seeing miraculous healings on a fairly regular basis! Blessed be! I am taking less insulin . . . I now know I probably won't need it. It's all shaking me free of the past program. Thank-you! Lots of Love! —Steph

My business is profitable in "these" times! —LeAnn

That regular Divine Opening is fifteen-twenty minutes of pure bliss that began to last longer and longer and longer. With much love and gratitude, —Teresa Anton, Pekin, Illinois

A warm tingly feeling spreads all through me, and in the morning when I wake, it's there again! Thank you so much for being there. —Elaine, Germany

I'm smiling too much; my husband doesn't know what to do with me! I have this amazing expectation that something big is about to happen . . . our financial/work headaches which were quite big now appear to be getting smaller and smaller. I am trusting Him in everything. What peace. Thank you, —Audrey, United Kingdom

Your work has the power of an atomic reactor. I was flooded with an incandescent internal light that was flooding thru me and the universe for quite a while. The next day I listened to one of the Diving In audios. I thought I was beaming off enough light to keep the east coast lit up for the remainder of the year. My dog was blissfully rolled over on her back and in sheer delight. She told me in doggie Yiddish, "who knew this Lola had such power, and from a recording no less." She sends ten energy licks of love for your face! I couldn't even sleep last night. —Love, Mark

Just wanted to share my appreciation of Divine Openings and say thanks. I have been reading the book, taking the course on-line and recently received a Divine Opening via conference call. VA vat voom! Divine Openings has had such a powerful and yet subtle, gentle impact on my life. I used to dip down quite frequently and since coming to the website that first time, I find myself each day, staying steady or experiencing joy and more joy. —Laura

I am continuing reading your book and I am reading it slowly as well as trying my best to put into practice simultaneously whatsoever I read. I do feel that I am making a lot of progress, I feel my peacefulness is deepening and always happy all the time and very much energized and also, I feel a mild blissful current running in my body most of the time. Love and Peace, —A. Punjabi, Philippines

Thank you for entering my life. —Conny, Malaysia

I'm now at the beginning of the online course, Week 1 and I already love it! Thank you for making this course reachable for many of us throughout the world! —Natasha, Macedonia

The book is so very helpful. I had an incident this morning where I went into judgment and looked for the place in the book to learn how to be with and let emotions move through me. I made the request of the Divine and felt the compassion for myself and for others who get caught in it, and then I felt the release. It was just that simple. I do not even need to have a conversation with that person. Much Love, Many Blessings, —Cindy P, Austin, Texas

I can read your book only bits at a time because the energy is so strong. I have been developing my personal relationship with My Divine. I used to have that HUGE nebulous BIG SOURCE that was too big and abstract to contemplate as a personal friend. I do appreciate the 'structure' for my mind. —Beverly, United Kingdom

Every time I have sat down to email you in the last 5 weeks or so I kept remembering something else wonderful that's happening. James, software engineer, UK

You and your work continue to make such an enormous impact in my life. Though I've been on the "path" for about 30 years, I consider putting into practice what I learned from you the real start of my spiritual journey nine years ago. I am forever grateful to you. Blessings, Anand-Sara, teacher, California

I started Divine Openings by reading and re-reading the book then taking the online courses. Having lost my son five months before I was going through the darkest time of my life. I was touched by Grace when I found Lola Jones and Divine Openings -- I will be forever thankful for such a blessing. From that point on I turned out to be a different person and my life has changed since I was led to a place where I had never been before - there is Peace in here. Who I am now and who I was before Divine Openings are all the way two different dreams. My love to you, dear Lola and to all. Lena, New York

You and your teaching have been so incredible for me -- the answer to what I had been asking for years -- it is like a birthday present for me every day "opening" the gift of your website, your online classes, your webinars, your videos, your books. Thank you so much for the beautiful gift of YOU!! See you on the next webinar!" Jennifer Cochran

I had a very vivid angel vision after a Divine Opening from the book... a very clear picture of where the spirit of my son's dad is (who passed away)... of his soul being embraced by angel wings. I've never experienced anything like that and it brings such a feeling of peace. Thank you so much! I'm re-reading your book too. Positive energy is spreading to my family and clients! Kelly, counselor, Austin, TX

Hi Lola, this is Sue from way down under in Australia. After my second Divine Opening, holy cow I felt a full range of emotions and the hairball I coughed up was HUGE. I went into a very dark place and I was angry, depressed, sad, lonely, and I was questioning everything and so much doubt crept in, the funny thing was while I was saying out loud "this is all crap, why am I bothering, etc, etc I found myself speaking to the Divine within ....Phew! I sobbed and swore and paced around my house and then I did your Diving In process. I asked the Divine to pull me up by the hand and guide me through the tough stuff, and for the next few days my emotions were all over the place ... and then all of a sudden, the most beautiful sense of peace came over me and now I am feeling so happy and my cheeky, funny, silly child within has come out to play! Cool, I'm having fun! —Sue, Australia

The book has been everything I was looking for and more. So much has happened in the sixty days since opening it the first time that it would be virtually impossible to tell you everything. —Sallie B.

Awareness's of how I've been resistant to receiving came up strongly. I asked God to soften that in me and then that "opening download" happened again immediately, and He told me, held me and showed me exactly what to do . . . I just experienced God in a much more intense way than ever before. I surrendered more than before and experienced a surging need to write even as I sobbed and yawned and released. I started in my journal and God wrote back. I've never experienced automatic writing before—what an awesome experience. Thank you for helping me remember my way Home as I'd gotten lost lately, and for helping me to access this amazing connection consciously in my daily life instead of just on retreats. Blessings to you, —Michelle Wolff

I felt a presence in the room, and could feel something 'opening', I can't exactly explain what opened up in me, but my more expensive work started selling. I sold one of my $2000 art pieces and the woman ordered two custom lamps too. —A. Broesche, Burnet, TX

My dog is so much better since the Divine Healing you sent. She had calcium deposits in her hips and was having difficulty getting around. Now, instead of limping and moaning and lying around on the floor and at the bottom of stairs she was avoiding, she is back to her old self—running, jumping on and off the furniture, going up and down stairs, and chasing her pal Shortie! We are overwhelmed with gratitude. Everyone who hasn't yet fallen in love with you, dear Lola, will, when they get your spirit, mind, body beauty treatment! —Erin, New Hope, Pennsylvania

I am focusing more powerfully at school. I can't describe the feeling I have when I connect with God now. I have no words for it. If I catch myself telling myself unproductive stories, I stop now. It is working. —Everett, high-school student, Pennsylvania

I just had what was probably the most incredible weekend of my adult life. I performed some of my music and was deeply heard. I received so much validation, encouragement———it was almost scary. My body is also changing, opening up, healing. I am so blessed by all of the synchronicity in my life right now. Gratitude to you, sweet Lola, my cup runneth over. —Martha P., Georgetown, Texas.

I was hoping for some relief from the longstanding intense pain in my leg . . . I felt a tingling in my leg during the session, and the pain eased somewhat. Over the next few days, it became increasingly better, and is almost gone. I also felt some tingling in my injured shoulder. I had become resigned to that residual aching and restricted movement. That pain has gone, and I am able to move it much easier. I am so grateful. Sharon, The Woodlands, Texas

I couldn't feel my body anymore and I lifted up out of it. I've always wanted to do this and have meditated for years trying to. When it was over and I was back, I felt so good I didn't want to move, so I sat there for a long time. —Randy, Harlingen, Texas

Most places where I go or work are gradually raising in vibration, a few people at a time, even with the economy and oil prices. —George Phon, commercial electrician, California

After the first session, my endometriosis started healing. It's a miracle for me and I can hardly believe it's happening. I have felt generally at ease all week, and for the first time in years my mind is not making up stories about what could go wrong. —Michele, Austin, Texas

I have been seeing myself from outside my own body, and at first not recognizing it as me. I am in bliss much of the time, quietly smiling. Things just don't bother me. I am starting to exercise and take better care of myself. —Cindy, Houston, Texas

Three years ago, I lost everything, husband, house, career... and although life went on and friends took care of me, I would wake up in anxiety every morning. The morning after my first Divine Opening, I woke feeling calm and light. I kept waiting to see if the anxiety would strike, but it hasn't come back. —Lynn A., Austin, Texas

THAT is good stuff! I felt tension in my shoulder, jaw, and heart area release, and my head felt as if it was literally expanding. Things are getting wild. Much joy. XOXO. —Laura Graf, Singer, Austin, Texas
My seminars and treatments go easier and give both clients and myself more healing and pleasure, therefore filled up very well and expanded to Austria and South Africa even. My husband's work became more fun and better paid. We used to live (the five of us, I have three children) in a seventy-four square-meter flat and drive an eighteen-year-old car. Now we drive a five-year-old car with seven seats (so much space!) and live on 146 square meters with a stunning, big garden and

neighbors better than we could have possibly dreamed them! We still walk through this beautiful, amazing house with our mouths open and stroll through the garden raving daily. And money, the major issue before, just keeps streaming in! Apart from these changes, I laugh a lot more, feel more peace, more serenity, more power, more love—I sometimes feel bursting of it all, it is so wonderful. I call it stretching the love and happiness muscles. Lots of love, —Gabriele, Germany

In thousands of emails from readers and participants in more than forty live retreats I've heard it all—spontaneous openings in love and relationship, happiness for no reason, financial breakthroughs, oneness with God, quieter mind. Hidden talents emerge, creativity explodes. Fears, worries, old blocks, limitations, and stresses melt. Defenses and old hurts are dropped, relationships are renewed, and love returns. New love is found. New lives are begun. Don't compare your experiences to others' experiences, because yours will be unique and perfect for you. The most subtle experiences, like most of mine are, can be the most powerful and fulfilling.

The Divine does the heavy lifting. Your job is to stay out of the way.

I Am a "Specialist"

WHEN I WANT computer help, I go to a computer specialist. I ask within and get guidance on who to call or where to look, but I do let humans help me. Sometimes the computer fixes itself when I get back in alignment, but many times a solution comes through a specialist—a person, book, website, or thing.

I am a specialist in evolution. New, raw, evolutionary waves of Energy/Light/Intelligence "vibrate me." They are not verbal and could never be fully explained verbally—they stream in constantly, some through untranslatable abstract dreams. I am a natural transformer and translator who makes the Energy/Light/Intelligence accessible for other humans, especially in practical life applications. Most of the results of Divine Openings occur vibrationally, although the words do help the conscious mind keep up and get on board. That's as much as I need to know about it. I care nothing for esoteric discourse or theory. If it doesn't help people practically, it's utterly uninteresting to me.

Each of us has our own genius. You are a genius or specialist at something, and Divine Openings helps you discover and unfold it. So while I think it's ideal for you to become primarily inner-guided, I'm a specialist who can catalyze your awakening, speed and smooth the process, and support it ongoingly if you need or want that. I'm a specialist in bringing Heaven to Earth, bringing it down to practical, everyday life rather than just showing you how to float around in the spiritual realms. I won't tell you what you should do, or how you should live after your awakening—I just point to the door marked "Freedom," you walk through, and then it's your world to create however you wish!

How to Have a Great Start and Get the Maximum

YOU CREATED ME because you want to feel better, live life more fully, and have more of your heart's desires. You've wanted so many changes in your life for so long, and now you're here on the threshold. Welcome home! Here are some suggestions for an ease-filled beginning:

Let go of the need to mentally figure it out. The mind cannot fathom Divine Openings, and would try to stuff it into some existing category that shrinks it. Divine Openings is *beyond words and concepts*.

Commit to play with, feel, and experience each piece rather than just reading. Practice each thing you read that very week in your daily life. Don't make it work, make it play. That's how you really assimilate it. Go for it with all your heart—but gently, softly, and in no rush—step by easy step.

Those with decades of spiritual experience benefit from making a decision to become beginners again. A beginner's mind is open, empty, not so full of concepts. I still live curious and willing to evolve. The moment I think I know it all I am fossilized.

When you are "advanced" it helps to be extra mindful: if you hear your mind say, "I already knew that"—STOP! Open to the possibility a higher, next-level truth. Are you living it 100%? How could you get it at a new, deeper level? If you want it all, let go of everything you know. Ditch the second-hand concepts, cliché New Age truisms, and all that stuff someone told you or some book said. Open up a large empty space for *direct knowing from within*. Come to Divine Openings with the curious, eager, and open mind of a child. Then Heaven is not far away.

You may have searched for so long that searching became a lifestyle, a preoccupation, an end in itself, and the original reason for it was forgotten. Seeking addiction prevents enlightenment. You may have become discouraged, weary, or felt that the search would never end. Now you can *experience The Presence* instead of seeking The Presence.

Enjoy the ride, open your arms wide, relax your grip on the steering wheel, and paradoxically everything will come faster. Some of you will find yourself feeling noticeably lighter in a week, many more will in a month, all of you will notice a big difference in a year if you commit, enjoy, and don't dilute it. You'll see people around you transforming as you do.

You have Free Will. Even Grace cannot and should not take that away. You come to Divine Openings with varying degrees of willingness and openness. Some of you soften and let go quickly—some more gradually. Let go of everything that holds you back. Strong resistance to feeling slows you down, but don't worry—*it does not stop you.*

My intention is for you to discover your own main line to your Source. Sure, many people in your life have gifts for you. They say or offer something at just the right time. They open doors for you, or add richness to your experience. The Divine Life Force lives and expresses through all of us. Be open-minded, but be very picky about what you let in—there's so much stuff out there that doesn't work, that isn't helpful and can pull you off track. Surround yourself with uplifting people, things, events as much as you can. If you don't have a Divine Openings community yet, many have started a book study group for a few family and friends. But if anything tempts you to give your power away to anything outside you, think carefully, it is a crucial choice. Divine Openings keeps guiding you back inside yourself, over and over.

You can begin to let The Divine do the heavy lifting now.

MARK THIS MOMENT – You will quickly forget your old reality, so take notes now!

Today's date _____

Write what you want—the whole list, including what you think is impossible. What you want to let in and *how you want to feel.* Tuck in extra sheets if you need to.

What you want that you've "worked at" but hasn't happened. How will you FEEL?

What your current challenges are. How will you FEEL when they're resolved?

What you want to let go of. How will you FEEL when you're free of it?

Sign and date to commemorate this new beginning: _____ _____

FOLLOW UP: At three, six, and twelve months, review what you originally wrote, and notice the changes in your life. Note how the things you wanted change as you lived into your authentic Self. One thing is certain—no matter how it plays out, or in what form, you can have what your *heart* has truly desired for so long.

Write how you feel at three months:

Write at six months, focusing on how you now FEEL:

At twelve months, focusing on how you now FEEL:

What has happened in your physical world at one year?

How has what you thought you wanted now changed? How has the value of feeling good changed for you?

Dancing Lessons From God

WHEN I TOLD a friend this book was about what happens when the small self gets in the back seat and the Large Self drives, he teased, "So then the story will have some exciting car chases and rollovers?" I laughed, "Life is more like a *drama-free zone* once the Large Self is driving." Once you Dive into your own true Being and start living as your Large Self, instead of drama you'll have adventures you enjoy and create on purpose.

My life wasn't always drama-free.

The desire to do what I do now was born when I first laid eyes on an enlightened master, my first teacher, in 1985. "But get real," I told myself, "you can never be what he is." My secret dream, too unbelievable to share with anyone, was to write a book that could change people's lives, even in my absence. The years went by and I forgot my "foolish" desire. If you had told me back then, in the thick of a rollercoaster life of unpredictable ups and downs, that nineteen years later I would indeed write that book, it would've felt hopelessly out of reach for me—another universe.

The best things in my life have always come naturally, not as a product of the mind alone. Our Large, Unlimited Self knows what we want more than we ourselves know, and the best form in which to deliver it. But I still didn't completely let go and let my Large Self do the work until I was past fifty, when Divine Openings arrived. Now I set no goals, yet things move faster, and there's more happiness than ever.

The September 11, 2001 terrorist attack coincided with my big mid-life hormone crash, and my lucrative corporate training and consulting career and all my motivation vaporized almost overnight. I stopped my spiritual teaching and counseling as well. I told God I was sick to death of mere words and their limitations, and was soon guided to be an artist for two years to play in the creative silence and restore my soul. I thought, "I'm middle-aged and burned out. *I can't rebuild it again.*" But in the barren cold of winter, unseen underground forces are always at work, gathering, building. For some time I had sensed something big was coming—as usual, something I clearly could not plan for or predict. What came was beyond my wildest imaginings.

How I Learned to Be with What Is

BY MARCH 2006 I found myself on a flight to India, mysteriously compelled to spend twenty-one days in silence. For those twenty-one days I dived deep inside, direct to The Presence, having my own inner-guided retreat rather than following "the program." Frankly, India was never on my travel wish list. I've never studied eastern religion and was thoroughly uninterested in India before I was called from within to go,. I have no need or desire to go back. I know I've lived many past lives there, but now I know everything we need is right here, right now—always.

During that twenty-one days in solitude and silence, communing only with The Presence within, a profound ability to open people to Grace blossomed. Those three weeks were so delicious I scarcely noticed the hard concrete floors I sat upon, the tiny barracks beds in the dorm, and the awful food. Other people were there, but I didn't get to know any of them. My focus was 100% inward—I wasn't there to socialize—I was there to go within and end my outer dependence. While few of the others observed total silence, I did—and made only enough eye contact to avoid bumping into people in the dorm hallways. The absolute silence was profoundly and permanently transformative for me.

I did it for myself, not realizing at the time that it would fulfill my secret dream to transform lives with ease. My fervent desire was to go within without distraction, and commune only with The Presence. I embraced the opportunity fully, and it changed my life. In that sheltered, secluded environment, there was nothing else to do or attend to. I chose not to communicate with home by phone or email except on a couple of occasions when I emailed briefly to say I was alive and well.

What a deep respite it was—perhaps a once-in-a-lifetime opportunity to have three weeks to do nothing but commune with The Absolute. It was Heaven! It left me more relaxed than I'd ever been in my entire life. It has lasted in spite of the much busier schedule that I now have since the success of Divine Openings, with many events, courses, music, and art projects., as well as people to manage.

The chronic tension and anxiety I carried my whole life disappeared permanently. If I get stressed, I notice it, breathe to soften into it, and it leaves, because my body is awake and alive with Intelligent consciousness. It corrects itself with just a little awareness, or with a little nudge from body-work or exercise. Energy work from someone else becomes unnecessary once you learn how to manage and move your own energy.

Emotions of every kind rippled through me one after the other during the twenty-one days. First, terror when my passport was taken away to a nearby town to be photocopied. I feared I'd never see my passport again. I lay awake terrified all night the first night, certain I'd be stranded in India if they lost it, but I sensed this drama merely triggered decades of old anxieties. It was an invitation for me to experience the fear fully, without trying to fix it or make it go away, and so reclaim that energy and raise the vibration of it.

By the second day the fear was bearable, by the third day it was a non-issue, and I actually laughed as my passport was handed back to me on the fourth day, long after they had said I'd get it back.

Emotion came in waves, flowing through me and the others, often without any reason. Causeless joy, causeless anger, sadness without content. Tears came, and left again just as suddenly. Much of what we feel may not even ours—it's the fear or sadness of humanity. We pick it up from Ancient Mind, a massive and powerful collective thought form. Every thought that has ever been thought is still accessible. We pick up Ancient Mind's vibrations, and then we attract more of that vibration, and on it goes, down through the generations. You will notice and raise those Ancient Mind vibrations as you progress through the book.

Much of what runs us is an ancient, flawed software we inherited.
Divine Openings upgrades it.

Waves of angst about a past relationship crashed over me as I bobbed in a sea of fear, sadness, and grief on another day. I had been in such a steady, happy place back at home and knew the importance of feeling good, but there were obviously blind spots I'd not been aware of—now they were up in my face! I'd not been able to even identify them before, much less change them, and now they came roaring to the surface.

Sometimes I got lost in inner questions and doubts that spun crazily in my mind, "What am I doing here? I feel so much worse than before I came!" Once I remembered to simply feel and allow the feelings, fears I hadn't been able to overcome in all my years on the spiritual and personal development path simply resolved, raising my vibration to peace, with moments of bliss. I found that any feeling, fully experienced, dissolved, that as lower energy rises to a higher frequency, *that power is reclaimed* and becomes available for productive uses. Then I knew deep down I was on track. I knew the silence would give me the total freedom I sought. It did, and it has lasted.

As I learned to lay it all down and let go, I tapped into Grace, which does for us that we cannot do for ourselves. Every powerful agent of The Divine that has walked the planet gave us a gift of Grace— to lift us up in ways that our own human efforts simply couldn't do.

With Grace assistance, when you can fully embrace even one or two core emotions, and allow and accept them, they rise in frequency. All emotions are soon mastered once you lose your resistance to allowing feelings to move freely. The backlog that bogged us down rises with them. Endless processing of issues gives way to simply flowing feelings in real time.

Gone are the days when you had to work individually through every emotion, issue, and trauma you'd ever experienced in your past! Thank God that old paradigm of processing issues one at a time, layer after layer forever *is over*. Divine Openings collects all the threads together and raises vibrations en masse, and then you'll simply do your best to stay current with what arises from then on.

Surprisingly, the emotion I struggled with longest was anger at those people who whispered with other people in our dorm room and in the dining hall, disturbing my delicious sacred silence. I knew they were terrified of the silence and of facing themselves in it, but I wanted them to be quiet and let *me* enjoy it. And how dare they break the rules! This indignation was odd; I'm not a rule follower myself. I wrestled with my harsh judgment of them longest and hardest of all, while the "big life issues" shifted with total ease!

Judgment is a deeply ingrained human habit. Most religions have steeped us in it. Finally I could just be present with my judgment, witness it, and let it be. "So I'm judging them as weak and inconsiderate because they're wasting their precious time here. So be it!" Then it dissolved and I looked at them with understanding and compassion. Voila!

As each wave of every imaginable emotion passed, I felt steadily more able to stand in them un-fazed, increasingly opened. Fearing no emotion, I became free. A new hope began to sprout in the hard, parched ground of my many years of endless seeking and growing discouragement. This was different than anything before it. I felt a depth and a certainty within myself begin to open up. My greatest desire was to become totally inner directed, free of the need to go to others for answers and healing—to have my own main line to The Divine. In the deep, rich, increasingly thought-free silence, that wish was coming true.

As I let go and let energy move, my vibration rose from hope to joy to ecstasy, with the occasional dip into feelings we call negative. I began to accept and welcome even those unpleasant or painful feelings, to appreciate them as "temporary experiences" with a valuable gift for me.

Equanimity and acceptance of all feelings ended the emotional rollercoaster ride I'd been on my entire life—a ride I thought I was stuck on forever. Equanimity is, quite simply, accepting what is. A miracle happened when I stopped resisting and trying to fix or change emotions and simply experienced them with soft acceptance: they moved with ease.

Although a few days were intensely difficult, overall it was beautiful and awe-inspiring. A few minutes of bitter tears, an hour of deep pain, or a few days of fear or anger were always followed by profound peace or even bliss. As vibrations were fully experienced—watching myself experience them without identifying them as me—without labeling them as good or bad or running from them, they always rose into the higher and finer vibration of my Large Self. Those low feelings weren't me! How fascinating to experience that, cradled securely in the arms of The Divine.

I relaxed further once I saw the possibilities. As long as I didn't resist, I was soon freed. Fear of feeling and resistance to feeling cause more suffering than the original feeling itself! I saw other people resisting and not getting this, and yes they did suffer. Those who resisted hard, about 80% of the people, got physically ill. I would never again would be afraid of any feeling. This has resulted in a remarkable, lasting peace.

Back at home I was soon able to be as centered and productive while feeling grief as while feeling ecstasy, whereas before, a strong negative feeling could derail my productivity and happiness for months or years at a time. There was now a certainty deep within me that popping back up to happiness was natural and inevitable—that anything except happiness was merely a *temporary* separation from my Large Self. All I had to do was relax and let go, soften into the feeling, to return gently to my Large Self.

After the delicious twenty-one days, I was for the first time in my life no longer at the effect of outside circumstances, other people, negative emotions, the world, the economy, or the troubles of the world. Solid in my center, nothing brought me down for long. I felt light, transparent, and unsinkable.

What you can't be with rules you. Be with what is and you are free.

Energy and Emotion Must Move

EMOTION AND ENERGY are supposed to move and flow through us. When emotion or energy is resisted and can't move, we get out of sync with the Flow of Life. Every disease or malady can be traced back to stress or stagnant energy that was not allowed to move freely.

Too many spiritual people try to avoid lower emotions, magically transcend them, make them go away with sessions or modalities, or deny them. They want to avoid any "bad" lower emotions and leap straight up into higher ones. I coined the now-common term "spiritual bypass." Interestingly, spiritual development is stunted until you deal with the very human realm of emotions. Enlightenment requires fully embracing the whole human experience, fully embodying the physical—not rising above it or escaping it. As enlightened humans, we're bringing Heaven to Earth, not looking for a fast pass out of here.

When we try to cling to positive feelings or experiences, we're operating as if there is a scarcity of them. When we realize that there is an endless supply there is no need to try to freeze them and keep them. Let them flow. Stop trying to hold onto positive emotions or experiences, or trying to push away negative emotions or experiences, since doing either is trying to stop something that is innately designed to flow. Nature moves. Energy moves.

It's your birthday party and you open a fabulous gift: you savor it, you pass it around and enjoy it as long as you can, but the next gift you open will be different. It won't be the same as that one, but you can enjoy the next one too, and then move on to the next gift, and the next. Experiences are like that. Blissful or painful they come and go, and there will be more. Source provides an endless supply of delights and experiences, and when we're open and relaxed, each one gets sweeter than the last, eternally.

Don't hold onto the gift.
Hold onto The Giver.

I was soon able to "be with" and allow any negative thought or emotion to move on through me within minutes of its arising, no matter how heavy, how old, or how strong. Eventually everything I felt or thought gently passed, leaving at the very least peace, emptiness, and a quiet, still mind in its wake, and at the very best, bliss. It was hugely freeing.

Now emotions that used to sink me for months or years can literally explode into multi-colored bliss inside me within minutes. At the bottom of everything is bliss. At my core is bliss. This is no surprise once you realize that your Large Self experiences only bliss. When you're experiencing something less, you're just not fully in alignment with your Large Self. You've wandered off course and gotten separated from the Oneness, the Flow of Life. Soon you'll know how to get back home easily. You'll know the address of Grace.

You can easily witness or observe yourself "having" emotions without getting mired "in" them. Nothing will ever be as gripping as it used to be. Students tell me nothing bothers them for long anymore. I feel everything, but I cannot imagine ever being terribly devastated again by anything.

As resistance to "what is" softened and eventually relaxed, as all that recovered energy lit me up, all my senses opened up, and I began to feel everything with a delicious new intensity. Even my sense of smell improved. I felt wide open and wide-eyed, like a new baby. With decades of backlogged lower vibration now moved in a relatively short time, I felt light as a feather, and the predominant feeling was happiness without any cause.

Within nine months of coming home from India, I stabilized, established a local Divine Openings following, and wrote this book. Many lifetimes of being an enlightener were reactivated in that silence, enabling me to activate the awakening process in others and change their lives—to relieve emotional, mental, spiritual and physical suffering without work and processing. Life issues, even things people have worked on for decades, now resolve easily. For the advanced, enlightenment is deepened.

Some of the teaching offered in the twenty-one days was a good fit for me; the rest did not resonate with me at all, especially the giving of all the power to the gurus. I've done this work in many previous lives, so it was more of a remembering than learning. It was quickly clear after the retreat that I would go my own way and continue my evolution through Divine guidance and direct knowing. The power increased without the buffer of the teachers. A passion arose: to find ways to help people "go direct" to their inner source.

I found that in addition to receiving Grace, students need a step by step system to retrain their unruly minds. It's as if part of them has become enlightened, while the mind still clings to old structures, as if clinging to a tree in a flood. An effective method of conscious mind retraining was absent in the organization in India, and many still struggled afterward in their daily lives, or kept seeking—not the result I wanted from my teaching. I was guided to create ways to support the mind during the awakening process, to apply enlightenment to everyday practical life, and sustain it.

Some of what I now teach came to me intuitively as long as twenty years ago, and some is influenced by beloved past teachers. Most comes from The Presence Within expressing through me. Giving this gift of Grace requires no effort, thought, study, or work. The less I "do" the better—Grace does most of the work. I felt I had finally come home after wandering in the desert—home to my own heart, my own Source.

I joke about my science fiction life, but the funny thing is, now it seems quite normal. Many of my students have much wilder mystical experiences than I do.

Different people are drawn to different teachers, because different teachers are called to say it in different ways. Divine Openings of course isn't the only way, but it works better than anything I've ever known, it ended my seeking, and has awakened many all over the world. I offer it in that spirit.

I offered the first Five-Day Retreat, and people registered for it without question. Going to India isn't a necessary element—I can take people into the silence anywhere in the world, anytime, and get them to that deep place much faster. It is necessary to get people away from their "normal reality" for those five days, so they have nothing else to do or attend to, and their focus is singular.

The first few years I gave Divine Openings, the intense Energy/Light/Intelligence flowing through me dominated my entire being, challenging my nervous system's capacity to handle it. I couldn't do anything else for about two weeks before, during, and after the Five-Day Retreats (my left brain barely worked.) All of my mind, body, and spirit's resources were used, much as running a very large program on your computer doesn't allow you to run other programs at the same time. It wasn't hard, it just *required everything I had*.

It was similar to being wired for 110 volts of electricity, and trying to run 220 volts. Now, the continual new incoming Energy/Light/Intelligence is more easily assimilated as my "wiring" continues to be upgraded, as yours will be. I can now function more normally when leading retreats and initiating others, although my human self is somewhat "absent." Things do go great in my absence!

We'll dive deeper as we go, and I lay the foundation purposefully. Read slowly and let the energy prepare you step by step as you read and feel. Notice any impatience. If you're saying, "I'm advanced, so I can skip this part," *STOP!* That will cause you to miss important things. Slo-o-o-ow down! "The last shall be first, and the first shall be last," and "You must come as a little child" now make total sense to me. It means you must let go of all you *know* to go higher, to get into Heaven. That's what I deliberately did in my twenty-one days—*I let it all go—I got empty*.

I know you're getting eager! My stories are softening and preparing you to allow more of that ease and Grace for yourself—to get off the hamster wheel of emotional processing and endless working on yourself and just let it in. Soon I'll share the revolutionary foundational "how-to's" of Divine Openings with you.

First, I invite you into a big-picture perspective. This focus on emotions is going to pass, and you'll soon be living in a fresh, new reality with very little dramatic emotion. Tears are likely to be tears of joy. Once all the energy that used to be tied up in lower vibration is liberated, you begin using it to play and create—living fully—more powerful and free than you thought you could possibly be. Surprisingly, mastering your emotions is your ticket there. All the esoteric metaphysical studies in the world can't bypass mastering your emotions, which are your vibrational Instrument Panel.

What Divine Openings does is beyond healing, cleansing, clearing, energy work or therapy. It affects people permanently because they learn how to manage their own vibration. Divine Openings awakens people with pure Energy/Light/Intelligence. The planet, the sun, the Internet, computers, money, thought, rocks, the ocean, and you and me are made of Energy/Light/Intelligence, but many humans have been asleep and have let their frequency get distorted. They've bought disempowering beliefs from others and from society. As you awaken and vibrate with a pure, undistorted frequency that's in alignment with the Flow of Life, issues and problems disappear naturally, because they don't resonate with you anymore.

What's most real is invisible and can't be seen. Scientists have been dropping clues for us for at least fifty years that nothing is solid—but they can't explain why it acts and appears solid to us. What physicists have found is so fantastically surreal that many of them quickly "forget" what they saw, because the mind has difficulty accepting it.

The Non-Physical is the birthplace of all material and non-material manifestation, so Divine Openings puts more attention and focus on creating in the Non-Physical rather than working so hard on the physical level—the hardest, densest level at which to work. Each time this awareness drops more deeply into your knowing you become more free. Nothing is solid or unchangeable. Everything is born of pure possibility.

Millions of years ago, you were just a possibility.

The End of Effort

AS I EVOKE Divine Openings I completely let go to my Larger Self and let it use my body, mind, voice, and hands—all of me—while I relax into the blissful sensation of my "smaller self" being absent. There's no work or thinking. My trying to *do* or *know* too much would seriously diminish the power and results of it. Delicious, causeless tears of love and bliss might stream.

This Golden Age you are choosing to enter (whether others on the planet do or not) is the end of effort—a return to the easy, effortless flow of Life, a return to The Garden, where we're aligned with The Divine such that we are led in every moment, surely, swiftly, accurately to what we want and need. The "efforts" I make, and even my challenges, feel more like play, creativity, and productivity than what I used to think of as "work." I'll think my life is full of ease, then am surprised to find yet another level of ease. There is always *more*.

The light of the Divine has always been inside you; enlightenment restores the ability to see it. All your power is right here, right now. All you need to know is available here and now. Seeking too much intellectual knowledge is a mind trap—you can never get enough. I've never seen that liberate anyone— understanding and knowledge are the booby prize, the small self's way to keep us chasing after more, more, more information.

The passing age has been one of man exploring his own Free Will, guided by his logical mind instead of The Divine Intelligence within, buying into the illusion that the physical world is immutable and all-powerful—often at the cost of losing his own happiness and fulfillment. It's been a grand drama. We're proud of our struggles and suffering. We make heroes of those who were lost and then found, as any movie plot demonstrates. Struggle is highly valued and rewarded.

We have taken off in our airplanes and pointed straight into a strong headwind, straining our engines, pushing with all our might against the flow that would carry us with a fraction of the effort if we allowed it. If anyone were to say, "Ummm, you could just turn downwind and go with the natural flow of Grace," we might say, "But where's the glory in that? I'm strong. I want to succeed my way and prove it." And it is true that everyone from our parents to our clients and employers cheer us on when we work hard, when we struggle and fight, sweat and strain. "Good work! You're such a hard worker! You have such perseverance! You overcame adversity."

Here's the good news. Finally, we're remembering that most of the adversity we were so busy overcoming… was our own creation. Now as we get out of the way, there's so much less to overcome. We can use that energy for more pleasurable, proactive, rewarding adventures and creations.

The world can't be changed from the outside, but what's in each human can be awakened. No amount of teaching, policing, regulating, legislating, forcing, controlling, or punishing has succeeded in changing the world. Such a shift can only come from within. When people are governed by the heart and guided by their Inner Source, no external regulation is required.

Einstein said that no problem is solved from the same consciousness that created it. I show people how to stop trying to tackle problems solely on the physical plane, but instead, shift their consciousness before action. From this new perspective, often the old problem simply isn't there to solve anymore! An experience of mine illustrates this. I have to reach way back to find such a dramatic example of struggle. It's simply not a big part of my reality anymore.

Many years ago, when my vibration was a lot lower, a Houston lawyer decided not to pay me twenty-four thousand dollars he owed me. He knew I would probably sue him after many months of sending past due notices and calling his office to no avail. So he sued me first, which put him in control of a game at which he excelled. I was fearful, as I had invested months in the project and needed the money, and was afraid he'd sink me financially with the legal expenses he could force me to run up. I hired an attorney, went over and over the facts obsessively, made the Houston lawyer the bad guy, and laid awake nights quaking, obsessing over what to do and how terrified of him I was.

After about six months (I was a little slow back then) I finally turned it over to The Divine and asked for dream guidance. Soon I had a dream in which a formal, authoritative man in a tuxedo gave me the keys to a very large white automobile. It was so huge I could barely see over the steering wheel. As I drove out of the car lot, I stopped to ask the man questions. He simply waved me on, ordering, *"Just drive away."* I woke with a whole new perspective; in that dream my consciousness had been instantaneously adjusted to peace and wellbeing. From that day on, I never thought about the situation again except to recount the fantastic dream of the white car. I never made the Houston lawyer the bad guy again—I was resolved with him, compassionate to him and his own demons. I knew it was over long before there was a shred of physical evidence. Feeling a little better and vibrating a little higher always precede improvement in the physical world. I just "drove away" as directed, focused on other things, and moved ahead with life.

Just drive away.

I heard nothing for another six months. One day my attorney called with a settlement offer of five thousand dollars. I confidently said "no" and once again forgot about it. Months later, another call came, this time with a settlement offer for twelve-thousand dollars. This time I said yes, since the money would be timely, and it would all finally be over and resolved—that was worth thousands to me. In that past state of consciousness, that settlement was the best victory I could manage, and it was pretty good. In today's consciousness I would have said no to that settlement, confident that I would get it all or even more in time. Seldom do I find myself playing victim roles in this new consciousness, although victimhood is seductive because the victim gets to be right—the innocent *good guy*. You'll learn it's not worth it.

At each chapter throughout that saga, my way of dealing with it shifted with each elevation in consciousness, and as Einstein predicted, the solution existed in a completely different consciousness than the one in which the problem was created. My life is largely drama-free now, and I'm clear that I am the author of it all. Today and going forward, I'd be unlikely to manifest a lawsuit. That could only if I ignored or resisted my own guidance, or dropped into a lower vibration.

Today, when I urge students just to "just drive away" they get the metaphor. Do you need to clear, heal, process, analyze or fix your past? No. Just drive away, eyes forward. Don't worry about how—Divine Openings helps you do it. Just read on.

Reality is radically different at different levels of consciousness.

A certain way of Being produces certain kinds of doing, which produces vibrationally matching results. Most of the world throws action, time, money, and work at a problem instead of shifting the way of *being* that produced that problem in the first place. Action wasn't helping the legal problem—it was actually making it worse. Shifting my own *being* worked. When your business is not going well, an action approach would be to work harder and longer, get new employees, talk to creditors, or change your processes. But it would be more effective to *first* change the inner state that caused those past results. "Be" clearer, then you'll "do" more effective things, then you'll "have" better business results. Align energy and intention first—materialization follows.

"Be" it first, then you'll "do" different things, and then you'll "have" different results.

Some think if they had more money, things would go better, and then they could be happy. But that's backwards. That's "have, do, be." The reverse is true: when you commit to "be" happier and more centered, you "do" better, and then you "have" more money. I won't ask you to be a better "doer." You'll allow your true inner being to emerge until you are *being* your Large Self, then you'll allow your actions to flow naturally from that. Then your life and circumstances will shift to fit who you newly are. They must, and they will, without effort.

Since I mentioned money (a highly charged subject), consider this: happiness isn't dependent on how many dollars you have in the bank. When you're in the flow of life, what you need comes to you when you need it, sometimes even without needing money. When you feel secure in that knowing, the number of dollars you have stored up doesn't matter, although you may indeed find your savings growing. When

you don't feel secure, no amount of money makes you secure. You've seen millionaires who cannot rest or play, and are in constant fear of losing their millions. And they can lose it. You can feel completely secure with an empty checking account living in a tiny, cozy home when your relationship with your powerful Larger Self is secure.

Some of you will use your newly blossoming creativity and confidence to make lots of money. Some of you won't care so much about money once you're happy. It's your reality—your grand, creative experiment—and you get to choose. Once you're awake, you'll know what's true for *you*.

The phenomenon that we call our reality is not the solid, concrete thing we think it is. The translating mechanisms of our senses and our brain, and our collective agreement make it appear solid. My changes in my perception of the lawyer and the lawsuit produced changes in my physical reality. When you focus first on your consciousness, vibration, and state of being, material issues clear up.

Ten years ago I worked with people to change their thinking and their perception of life, and then their relationships would improve, their incomes would rise, and they were happier and more successful. That was all good, and it was leading-edge at the time, but there are now more profound ways to change reality. Divine Openings doesn't work on details and individual issues at all. It doesn't need to because it works at the meta-level (very big picture), and causes quantum evolutionary leaps at every level of your being simultaneously.

Divine Openings literally upgrades your software, reconnects DNA strands, switches on new evolutionary strands, restores lost connections to the earth and other dimensions, and activates your light body. Most people feel a tingling or expansive feeling after some number of Divine Openings from this book. Sit quietly after each Divine Opening to fully feel the nuances. You could *feel nothing* and still have dramatic changes in your life within weeks or months. Stop taking score. Notice what's better in your life. Journal only about your successes and what you appreciate, and limit talking about problems. You get more of what you focus on because your focus has enormous creative power in it.

Divine Openings opens you to Grace, without work.

If this sounds fantastic, there is more to come, much more. Momentum is on your side because evolution has been speeding up exponentially. Imagine if you were a cave man walking our streets, observing our computers, planes, and cars. It would be mind-boggling. More has happened in the last fifty years than formerly happened in many hundreds of generations. Even in the 1800s, could you have wrapped your mind around television, space travel, the Internet, cell phones, video conferencing, and jet airplanes? Our current reality will seem as primitive in retrospect as the cave man's seems to us now. From the limitations of today's consciousness we have no way to conceive of what's coming because that emerging future will be borne of tomorrow's consciousness.

These days you don't have to die to get a fresh new life. You can just start a new one right here—if you're willing to let go of even the best of what you knew before. I often muse about the many lives I've already lived in this body, and more are coming.

Divine Openings and I have continued to expand and evolve since those twenty-one days of silence. I even re-read this book, listen to my own audios, and take my own online courses because the Large Self

that writes and teaches is much wiser than the everyday me. Your Large Self will always be out ahead of your smaller, more limited self, calling you forward into your next level. Go and it feels good. Resist and it hurts. It's that simple.

I know many of you have a strong desire to make a difference on the planet, but take plenty of time get yourself completely free first. You can exhaust yourself doing it the old way. You're going to discover easier ways to change the world that you cannot now imagine—and there is no work involved. Fasten your seatbelts, place your tray tables in their upright and locked positions, and enjoy the ride.

It's an Experience, Not a Concept

JUST STUDYING AND TALKING about spiritual things is a barrier to inner knowing, because it remains merely mental without having real experiences. You're about to have a direct experience of The Presence within you. This invisible Larger aspect of You will soon become a normal everyday part of your life.

A Divine Opening can be activated in any number of ways. When I see people one to one I invoke Divine Openings by intention, or holding their hands, or I give astoundingly soothing Mother Hugs." When it's a large group I evoke the Divine Openings by intention from the front of the room, without touch. It's just as powerful. Divine Openings can also be activated through movement and art (as in this book), music, by phone, webinar. Divine Openings work by long distance too. Sometimes the group closes their eyes while Lola sings a song that carries the Divine Opening. In the Five-Day Silent Retreat, I give powerful initiations by gazing into your eyes: The Divine looking at The Divine.

You discover enlightenment only by experience—it's not something you can learn, figure out, or understand with the mind—so it's best to leave the mind out of it. Understanding is the booby prize. The most blissful states are experienced in No-Mind.

Divine Openings indeed activates or deepens your enlightenment by Grace, and helps you let more good into your life. It's all a matter of time, and the timing is for The Presence and you to decide. If you want results more quickly, soften your focus, read the book slowly and deliciously, but don't make it into work.

Intellectual, analytical people do better if they can let go of thinking, and feel everything instead. Simple villagers have become fully enlightened with one blessing by a master, because there was less mental clutter, and fewer ego constructs and spiritual pretenses to shed to restore that most simple, natural, and innocent state.

People sometimes tell me all the spiritual books they've read, the gurus they've lived or studied with. I'll teasingly say, "Then why have you come to me? You don't need me." Then they confess they're still not happy or fulfilled, or it's not "working" in their practical lives. Perhaps they're still struggling with money, or emotions, self-worth, anxiety, or relationships. They've found that the mind cannot take you there no matter how many books you read and how much religious or spiritual knowledge you accumulate. Enlightenment can't be earned by hard work or service. You can't rush or control it. Nor can you get it by being good, doing good works, or "being spiritual."

Divine Grace can give it in a heartbeat.

Divine Openings doesn't fit in any "spiritual" box. To have the most pure, powerful, and authentic experience leave all your old concepts of God, religion, and spirituality behind. You wouldn't eat

secondhand food. Don't ingest second-hand experiences of God, no matter who said it. You'll move faster if you open up to pure experience, and let go of mind stuff. People ask why I got more than others did in that twenty-one days of silence. I'll share more later but one key was: "I was willing to get completely empty."

Mental and intellectual understanding is the booby prize.

Divine Openings so profoundly changes you, and so radically shifts reality, that one week after a huge challenge is resolved it's common for a student to strain to remember what the problem was. It was *that gone*. It happens often—people go on to their new reality and soon forget the old one. They get so busy living they don't have much interest in the past. You'll know you're free when there's no interest in retelling past dramas and problems. This is the new paradigm of living in the now. The hazy past seems unreal.

The Small Self Lets Go

SOME CALL IT the ego, but I call it the small self so you can see it fresh and not make it "bad." Small self is simply a more narrowly focused, less knowing aspect of us that thinks it is separate from God, other people, and Nature; it's the part that resists the Grace that would carry us with ease. It is fearful, scarcity-oriented, defensive, habit-driven, and has created all kinds of compensatory strategies to protect against things that it itself has created. It believes that life is basically a struggle against something "out there."

Don't resist that smaller self or make it wrong—embrace it tenderly and talk to it soothingly as you would a fearful younger sibling.

When we rely only on our senses and those things we can see, feel, touch, smell and taste, we are an isolated small self, like an astronaut would be if there was no Command Central back in Houston to hold the Larger view and give guidance. He'd be lost, adrift, and all alone out in space. When we let go to the greater guidance of our Large Self, we have our own Command Central.

Our Large Self never loses touch with that broader perspective—it knows the bigger picture of our lives, the world, the universe, and the other dimensions. Small self is the lesser part of us that allows us to narrow down and have the illusory experience of being separate, unique human individuals, but we're always encompassed by and enfolded in the greater Large Self. Any actual line between the Large and small self is imaginary.

Your small self goes through a process of letting go of its fears. As you embrace and soothe it, it gets in the back seat and enjoys the ride while the Large Self drives the bus. Life goes more smoothly and there is more ease and Grace in your life when the Large Self is in the driver's seat. The small self can know fleeting pleasures, but it can't know joy until it has relaxed into the care of the Large Self.

This book guides you as you awaken, so you may now relax. When the small self stops struggling and gets on the wave the Large Self has created, we enjoy surfing Life. The ride is for fun, not to get somewhere or prove your worth. You'll discover your worth is a given, and that The Presence wants you to be happy.

VERY IMPORTANT!

Please read carefully before proceeding:

I am an evolutionary agent of Divine Energy/Light/Intelligence and I use the words in this book, the art, my music, my intention, and other direct Non-Physical means to translate and convey it to you. The Grace energy and your allowing and experience of it are more important than the words.

EACH TIME YOU come to a work of art in the book, gaze at it to receive a Divine Opening. A casual glance at the art will not give you a Divine Opening if you don't intend it. Each Divine Opening "expands your pipes," and opens you to let in more Grace.

- Wait at least two weeks between Divine Openings. More and faster is *not better*.. Each Divine Opening needs time to integrate and unfold fully before adding new energy. In general, slow down *everywhere* in your life to feel more, and paradoxically, evolve faster.

- Pregnant women past the second trimester may not receive Divine Openings until after delivery of the baby. Just read the book and intend the art to give you Divine Mother Hugs instead.

- Those with serious mental disorders should receive sessions before doing Divine Openings.

- Alcohol or mood altering drugs of any type interfere with your brain and feelings. Those with substance addictions may need additional Divine Openings help. See resources at back of book.

- Divine Openings are for those eighteen years or older. Those under eighteen can intend to receive Divine Mother Hugs from the book to help them develop and succeed in life.

- Receive only one Divine Opening every two weeks from any source. *"Advanced" people are no exception*. More is NOT better. The point is to enjoy! Don't speed up the energy faster than you can release resistance to it. You can read past a Divine Opening and come back and do it later.

- Each Divine Opening experience is different, so don't compare them, or have any expectations. If you don't feel anything, things are happening below your threshold of perception.

The awakening of Divine Intelligence within you automatically resolves anything it stirs up very quickly if you will soften around the feeling, dismiss judgment, and allow the feeling to be. Don't try to make any feelings that arise go away for they are valuable messengers that serve you! Resisting lower feelings got you where you are, and embracing them will take you to a realm of self-empowerment beyond your highest expectations. Be with and embrace all feelings softly, sweetly, kindly, and they will move up and resolve faster.

Never try to relieve or "fix" the after-effects of a Divine Opening—that interferes with this self-resolving process that needs no help at all.

Divine Opening

YOUR FIRST DIVINE OPENING is a special occasion that formally initiates you to enlightenment, or opens a new level. Take a moment now to review where you have been in your life, soften around and say goodbye to the past. You could offer appreciation for the Grace you are about to allow in.

Gaze gently at the work of art for about two minutes. Get out of the way. Simply allow Divine Grace to do it all. Then close your eyes, lie down, and rest for fifteen minutes or longer.

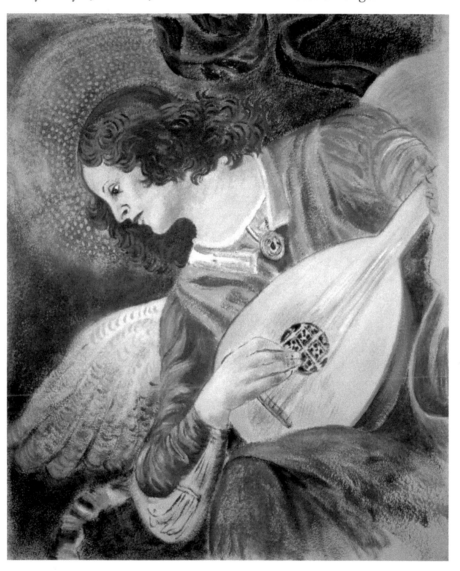

Figure 1—Angel, *a five foot mural by Lola Jones,*
her interpretation after Italian master Mellozo da Forli's Angel With Lute

After Your First Divine Opening

NOW YOU HAVE had your first Divine Opening, an initiation to enlightenment, or a deepening of your enlightenment. It works on the subtle planes. Regardless of how much or how little you can feel it, *it works on you just the same.* It is cumulative, and the effect builds with each successive Divine Opening.

Sometimes you feel nothing special, and then remarkable changes start occurring in the following weeks, in your body, mind, and feelings—in your life—and even in the people around you. Take care to notice and appreciate *every little wonderful thing that occurs.* Journal to yourself about your progress, and if you wish, share your successes at celebrate@lolajones.com or support@DivineOpeningsGermany.com.

Your Large Self designed your experience just for you, so rather than comparing it to someone else's or to something you read, appreciate *your* experience. Let go of expectations and judgments. No two Divine Openings are alike, so don't expect the same one to happen ever again. Let go of the last experience, and be open to new ones each time—as in Life! While live, in-person, webinar or phone Divine Openings are usually more intense, we hear many dramatic exceptions to that from readers. Subtle is just as powerful.

Each Divine Opening works on you intensely for weeks, months, and years, so notice and appreciate everything that happens in your inner and outer world, even those things you don't yet understand. Your life will forever be affected, made easier, and eventually it all makes sense.

You won't need a Divine Opening every two weeks forever. You'll soon access this Grace state by intention, and live in that state of Grace and flow more and more of the time. Most modalities are about clearing, fixing you, or making the feelings or the pain go away, but Divine Openings shows you how tap into your own inner source, where you find that there was never anything wrong with you.

You could benefit from body work, massage, Rolfing, Feldenkrais, yoga, chiropractic, acupuncture, music, dancing, and exercise to help the slower, denser physical self to soften, let go, and allow the flow. Energy work, most other modalities, and non-Divine Openings counseling contradict this energy and slows your progress.

Enjoy. Because it's all about joy.

Hitting a Speed Bump

LET'S COVER THIS now that you've had your first Divine Opening. People are conditioned to take unwanted emotions too seriously, so I came up with a benign and humorous term to lighten it up: "coughing up a hairball" (like cats do.) Some students called it "hitting a speed bump." The lighthearted names for it encourage people to lighten up about it—even laugh about it—and enjoy the movement more. It doesn't have to be heavy unless you resist it. Let your mantra be "it all moves softly and easily if I let it," and that eventually becomes your reality.

Everything does indeed shift more quickly if you don't resist, fight, or try to escape it. Fear, anxiety, worry, anger, uncontrollable rage, grief, depression, aggravation, jealousy, illness, fatigue, headache, nausea, digestive upsets, odd physical sensations, odd automatic body movements that you can't control, upsets with others, conflicts, financial scares, and setbacks—all of these can and do move easily!

Let it move with maximum ease, grace, and humor.

You're opening to embrace and appreciate the full range of emotions, from profound bliss to emotions you'd probably label as "unwanted." When you begin Divine Openings, you're asking Grace to raise your vibration, and as that happens, lower vibrational energies activate and begin to move upward en masse. Maybe in the past you'd get stuck in such lower feelings, but with the Grace-assistance of Divine Openings, they move quickly unless you resist feeling them.

We are deeply brainwashed that we must learn by suffering and progress by hard work—if you can let go of that, suffering isn't necessary *at all*. Just feel all feelings softly and let them move. Don't try to fix the feeling or make it go away, don't judge it or make it wrong, and you won't suffer.

Resistance turns pain into suffering.

After a Divine Opening you may feel blissful—or depressed, angry, enraged, or sad for no reason. Just be with it, soften into the feeling, and witness it, saying to yourself, "Oh, years of depressed energy is moving," or "Oh, it feels like sadness of decades is moving."

I'll remind you often, because when you're caught up in some feeling or situation you might forget that the emotion is perfect and try to fix it. Emotions are a sign things are moving, so appreciate and value all emotions and events–*all of them!* With Divine Openings, mountains of energies from decades and eons rise in vibration—en masse. Old beliefs and limitations crumble.

The best news is that as you feel a feeling, Divine Openings connects vast networks of similar vibrations, bundles them up, and moves them en masse. That's why you feel huge relief; you've liberated far more energy than you know.

These feelings and vibrations that arise are not new—they've been building up and have needed to move for a long time. They've been affecting your reality whether you knew about them or not. As you learn simple Divine Openings methods you soon welcome and even enjoy *all emotions* as they come to light and rise in vibration, bringing new freedom. Don't resist the feelings and you won't have to play them out the hard way, as unwanted events, conditions, people, stresses, or illnesses in your life.

Full body bliss—or lower energies moving up—welcome it all. We had a good laugh when a few students actually felt something physically scratchy in their throats like a hairball! Intend your awakening to happen with ease, Grace, and humor, and it can. Resist nothing, value and accept all feelings, and your awakening can be smoother. The bulk of your density usually lightens in the first few months or year of Divine Openings, *if you'll soften around those feelings and allow them*. It's fast. Those old days of endless processing are *over*. There is no work to do, just some focus and allowing.

I'll give you the tools you need—absorb and practice them one at a time. Help from Grace makes it possible with ease. As the years went by I noticed that as our Divine Openings collective became larger, everything became easier for the new people. It's as if you're standing on the shoulders of those who went before you and smoothed the way.

Let go of any belief in the value of suffering.
There is no value in suffering unless it's the only way you'll let yourself evolve.

Declare ease and Grace. I did, and I got it. You might actually *want* rivers of tears and drama so you have proof that "something big" is going on, but it isn't necessary. You can choose the easier way—I'll show you the steps. Once you say yes and your awakening begins, it's on cruise control with Grace driving. If things in your life break down, you weren't letting it happen any other way. Let them go to make room for better things.

Appreciate that the Larger Non-Physical aspect of you is right now moving those dense old postures, masks, strategies, defenses, structures, and patterns you had unconsciously created or picked up through the years. They were embedded down to your cells and atoms. Each Divine Opening dissolves what no longer serve you if you allow it. That old small-self density, the fearful illusion and pain your mind created, is not you, and as your vibration rises you become lighter, brighter, more radiant.

The Grace Piece, and the Conscious Mind Piece

Divine Openings is made up of 1.) the Grace piece and 2.) the conscious mind piece. The Grace piece is that gift that is not earned but is offered freely. As you learn to let more Grace in, it will do 90% of the work for you. The Divine Openings you'll receive through this book are pure Grace, and they work *on you* and *for you* in ways that you could not possibly do by human effort alone.

The conscious mind piece is your small part to do—it's only 10%, but it's vital. You apply the pleasurable conscious mind tools to make your best Free Will choices, and manage your mind so it's your servant rather than your master—your friend rather than your tormenter!

Long ago I found students transformed much more rapidly when they retrained their conscious minds in addition to receiving Divine Grace. The mind's fearful, change-resistant nature is soothed and calmed when your mind has some idea where your Large Self is leading you.

The conscious mind piece of Divine Openings was synthesized over several decades, from my dreams, my corporate courses, the work of Esther and Jerry Hicks and others, but most of it came from within. The Large Self and small self concept is something I developed decades ago for the corporate world. The most left-brained IBM software developers instantly recognized the practical value in distinguishing Large Self and the small self, without any spiritual context at all.

The conscious mind piece soon makes it easier to manage our small selves and fearful, runaway minds, but Grace still does most of the work. A woman told me recently, "The little devil inside my head is just gone and I don't even know why!" That was a gift of Grace. The Divine did the heavy lifting.

Now we delve into the conscious mind piece: using your mind and your Free Will wisely. It isn't work, it's just paying attention.

How to Navigate

NOW TO BEGIN to give you the fundamentals of steering your life and manifesting your desires. If you have difficulty allowing yourself to have the things you want in life, consider this: an enlightened person who is fulfilled and prosperous, and whose own needs are met, has more power and ability to make a difference in the world. Struggling to pay your bills and buy gas puts you in survival mode, and being in a low vibration isn't being the light unto the world that you could be.

Decades ago, for many years, I had a recurring dream in which I had a lit up, neon green "control panel" that I used to guide my spaceship. My hands fit perfectly into the indentions in it. Upon waking, it dissolved from my hands, even as I grasped desperately for it, feeling powerless. In later years, thank God, I found my long-lost control panel and gained constant access to it. I'm about to re-introduce you to *your* long-lost control panel.

On a recent flight, a TV screen in front of each seat showed our aircraft on a map of the world, alternating with flight statistics, so I always knew where we were, how far we were from the destination, the velocity, altitude, and direction of the flight. With the control panel back in my hands, life has become like that. It is no longer a blind flight, landing in some random place, wondering how I got there. Now I always know how I got there, and soon you will too.

Once you rediscover your marvelous control panel or "Instrument Panel," you will never again be confused, lost, or off-course for long. You will move surely toward the rendezvous point you desire, and you'll have plenty of time to change your route or altitude to avoid a collision or make your desired landing. You will never again be mystified by why anything happened, because you will see exactly how you navigated there, even if it was unintentional or unconscious. You'll know exactly where you are headed, how fast you are going to get there, and how it will feel once you get there. The past will make more sense, and the future will be easier to create.

Using my Instrument Panel and checking it constantly, I know exactly what I'm creating and where I am headed in any given moment. If I feel bad, I know I'm on a trajectory that will lead me to things I don't like. If I feel good, I know the destination will feel good.

Your Instrument Panel

FOR YEARS WE were told that our thoughts create our reality—that we get what we think about. No wonder we got so frustrated when it didn't always work. We didn't have our Instrument Panel, and we didn't have Grace doing 90% of the work.

Savor this section slowly. Even if you have read fifty books on Law of Attraction and think you already know this, there were secrets you weren't given, or key pieces left out.

Conscious *and* unconscious thoughts vibrate, and those vibrations radiate out from you like a radio tower broadcast. It attracts similar vibrations to you—people, places, and things that match your vibration. If you're broadcasting sadness, then more sad experiences, people, places, things are attracted to you. If you're *authentically* broadcasting happiness, and not spiritual bypassing, then more happy experiences, people, places and things are attracted to you.

Your Creator gave you feelings to help you know what vibrations you are broadcasting. Those feelings tell you how closely you are in alignment with your Large Self, or God Self, and are miraculous predictors of the reality you're creating next. If you are feeling the higher emotions about your desired destination you are in alignment with your Large Self, the larger-perspective you, on that subject. Being your Large Self feels better, and gets you where you want to go faster. You're feeling relaxed and allowing yourself to be guided and carried toward your desire.

Being your small self and feeling the lower emotions isn't *wrong*, it just isn't powerful and effective. Your Large Self is always at a high altitude, which means your Large Self always feels good, so if you feel good you can be sure you are in alignment with your Large Self. If you are feeling bad, you are simply out of alignment with your Large Self, and that is *supposed to feel bad!* Soon you will always know why your actions and plans are working or not working. You will always know where you are and which way is "up." With full use of your Instrument Panel, you'll always know whether you are in alignment with your Large Self—and if you're not, how to get back there.

Soon you'll know without a doubt whether you are headed toward your goal or away from it. Once you get re-calibrated to your Instrument Panel, you will never be "lost" again. Like the flight screen on my transatlantic voyage, it takes the mystery out of where you are, and how far you have yet to go. When you know where you are, it's easier to navigate to where you want to go in life.

Your Instrument Panel tells you where you currently are vibrationally *on a given subject*. You're at different levels on the Instrument Panel on different topics. For example: you might be at a high altitude about money and friends, and at a lower altitude about romantic relationship. Therefore your financial and social life is great but your romantic life is not so fulfilling. The Instrument Panel translates your feelings to altitude readings. It helps you remember what you knew when you were little. You knew how to read your feelings from your own Instrument Panel and naturally find your way up through the feelings, and to rise in altitude. A child, if allowed to do what it wants, naturally knows how to move up in altitude. But we lose touch with our own Instrument Panel over time by listening to other people instead of trusting our own knowing.

Since your Large Self vibrates up at the top of the Instrument Panel all the time, movement up the Instrument Panel is always movement toward your Large Self. At the top is POWER—not power over anyone else, but power over your own reality. When you're up there you have access to all the power of your Large Self—that's a lot of power. At the bottom is POWERLESSNESS.

The important thing is to feel what is "up" or "down" for *you* rather than following my description of the feelings to the letter. Up brings relief, down brings stress.

Before we introduce you to your powerfully effective Divine Openings Instrument Panel, clear your mind of any other modalities or emotional scales that may seem similar. Please approach Divine Openings and the Instrument Panel fresh, with the mind of a child, without preconceptions. We have evolved understanding of the hierarchy of emotions to a new level, and the boost of Grace makes it astonishingly simple to apply to your daily life for real transformation.

HOW TO USE IT IN YOUR LIFE: Print out the next two pages or download beautiful color copies in English or German at DivineOpenings.com/instrument-panel. Post them where you'll see them often. Notice where you are on the Instrument Panel several times a day. No judgment, blame, wrong making, or trying to change it. Just witness yourself compassionately.

Your Instrument Panel (Original)

Ecstasy   **YOU FEEL POWERFUL UP HERE.**

Joy, Bliss   You are your Large Self up here.

Direct Knowing, Empowerment   This energy is light, fast, flowing, un-resisted.

Freedom

Love, Appreciation

Passion, Eagerness, Enthusiasm

Happiness, Positive Expectation   **More Expansive Energy**

Belief

Optimism, Confidence, I Can Do It

Hopefulness, Seeing Possibilities, Curiosity

Self Esteem, Interest, Courage

Contentment, Relaxation, Emptiness

Acceptance, Boredom, I Don't Care ------- The resting zone, not exciting, but useful.

Pessimism, I Give Up

------------------ THE TIPPING POINT -------------------

Frustration, Aggravation, Impatience

Overwhelm, Stressed, Overwork   Much of society lives here and thinks it's normal.

Disappointment

Doubt, Confusion, Uncertainty

Worry, Negative expectation

Discouragement, I Cannot Do It, Fatigue

Anger --- A bridge to get your power/energy back.

Revenge

Hatred, Rage   **More Contracted Energy**

Jealousy, Desire That Feels Bad, Lack

Guilt, Blame, Projecting Negativity On Others

Fear   **YOU FEEL POWERLESS DOWN HERE.**

Sadness   The energy is slow, heavy, dense, resistant.

Grief, Depression   It's hard to hear your Large Self down here.

Shame, Unworthiness, Despair, Apathy

Every emotion on the Instrument Panel is Divine Energy at varying frequencies.

All emotions are valuable information. Appreciate them all!

Appreciation and love to Esther and Jerry Hicks, David R. Hawkins, and others whose emotional/consciousness scales helped me rediscover my long lost "control panel."

The Expanded Instrument Panel

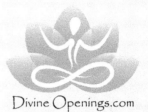

Divine Openings.com

Higher, Lighter Vibrations

Ecstasy, Joy, Bliss, Oneness, Knowing
Abundance, Empowerment, Worthiness
Freedom, Delight, Love, Appreciation, Harmony

Inner Guidance is Unmistakable
Inspiration, Wonder, Passion
Enthusiasm, Positive Expectation, Happiness
Belief, Confidence, Hopefulness
Seeing Possibilities, Curiosity
Self Esteem, Interest, Courage

The Tipping Point - Your Reality Starts to Change
Contentment, Relaxation, Acceptance, Boredom, Indifference
Emptiness, Quiet Mind, Pessimism, Giving Up

Resistance Loosens Up
Frustration, Impatience, Aggravation
Agitation, Nervousness, Overwhelm, Stress
Disappointment, Doubt, Confusion
Uncertainty, Can't Act
Worry, Insecurity, Negative Expectation
Discouragement, Quit, Tired

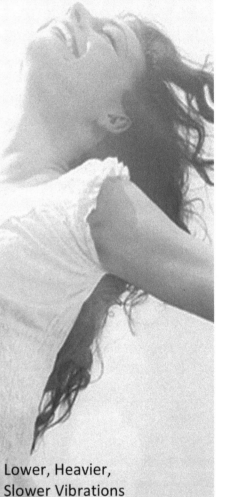

Lower, Heavier, Slower Vibrations

~ Anger - The Bridge ~
Revenge, Hatred, Rage, Jealousy
Addictions, Loneliness, Lack
Guilt, Blame
Fear, Sadness, Grief, Depression, Shame
Unworthiness, Despair, Powerless, Hopeless, Numb

Step by Step

IF YOU'RE LOW on the Instrument Panel on a particular subject in your life, it is creating a reality you don't want in that area of your life, but your job is not to get to ecstasy about it today. That's too much. Your job is to feel just a little bit better today and a little bit better tomorrow. You can do that. Some people get frustrated and quit when they can't get to joy today, or to skinny today, or to debt-free today. But think about it: would you expect a baby to learn to walk in one day or even one week? Would you expect to train for a marathon in one month after being out of shape for five years? NO! *Your success accelerates when you celebrate small steps.* Those small steps will take you there, and when you get there you'll be stable and you'll stay up there.

When you move "up" there's a slight feeling of relief, of regaining energy.

If you are feeling just a tiny bit better about money today, more money is coming in the days and weeks to follow. If you are feeling just a little bit better about your body today, a better body is coming. If you get discouraged, you split and contradict your energy, and your result is delayed because materialization follows vibration. Fretting adds resistance and contradicts your pure desire! Relax.

Make the most of the best, and the least of the worst.

You have different vibrations about various subjects your life. If you're in fear, despair, anger, frustration or any lower emotion in an area of your life, first soften and accept that "you are where you are." Just doing that moves you up the Instrument Panel to acceptance, to the middle, the Tipping Point! Then Grace and momentum helps you gain altitude slowly and steadily. Momentum is your friend once you get an upward trend going.

You don't even have to name the emotion—just feel it physically in your body and talk to your Large Self about how it feels physically. Naming the emotion is most useful is when, for instance, you notice that you've moved up from an *unworthy* feeling to *frustration*—that calls for a celebration. You suddenly appreciate that frustration, because while it still doesn't feel great, it's higher than unworthiness!

The general idea is to move up the Instrument Panel and feel better—even a little bit better helps. Rather than aiming for bliss today and failing, go for just a slightly better feeling, a slightly higher altitude. Stabilize there, and then move on up. You'll get up where your Large Self is eventually—but it's *easier to do it incrementally,* one step at a time, and it's longer lasting too.

There is no bad place to be on the Instrument Panel or as a human being. The Presence never judges where you are. Whenever you soften around a feeling and allow and make space for it, you're agreeing with The Presence who is already in that soft, accepting place.

Once you know how to navigate using your Instrument Panel, you can get anywhere you want to go from anywhere you are. If you're in Los Angeles and you'd rather live in New York, you'd get a map, get in your car and point it toward New York. You know it's a long journey, but you know you'll get there.

When you're familiar with your Instrument Panel you know where you are relative to your destination. By how you feel about it, and which way you're pointed, you can estimate how long it will be till you arrive. If you feel ecstatic about it, you'll be there soon. If you feel doubtful about it, it may take longer to arrive. If you're depressed about it, you're headed in the opposite direction.

Everything is Divine energy, but the vibratory rate of the emotions at the bottom of the Instrument Panel are at lower frequencies, relative to the un-resisted, higher, faster frequencies at the top. As you move up the Altimeter, vibration is faster, less dense. There's light, power, velocity, and vitality. As you move down, it's more sluggish and dense.

It's supposed to feel bad at the bottom of the Instrument Panel. It feels good to be at the top of the Instrument Panel because you're in alignment and agreement with your true, powerful Large Self. You obviously cannot get completely separated from your Large Self—that's impossible, you're part of it—but at the top of the Instrument Panel you're vibrating as your Large Self. Look at the Instrument Panel and *feel* in your body the levels of energy as they increase from the bottom upward. When you soften and allow feeling, that energy rises in frequency and gets more organized and Intelligent. Then you feel better, and soon things begin to go better. Resistance is simply contracted, tense energy, as opposed to soft, expansive, flowing, high vibrational energy.

The small self is by nature fearful, doubtful, and resistant, and has no interest in giving up control and softening into the flow, but your *intention* to feel good and put the Large Self in the driver's seat prevails over time. Be kind and compassionate with your small self—it's doing the best it can with its limited consciousness. It is fear-based, and so might resist anything unknown, just because it's new.

From your Large Self perspective, make the decision to soothe the small self and have it take a back seat. *Choose and decide* to let your Large Self fly the plane and orchestrate it all. It has a larger perspective and unlimited resources. It IS your Source.

The most exciting, empowering news is yet to come—we'll get there one step at a time.

Now you can begin to allow your Large Self to fly the plane.

APPLY IT TO YOUR LIFE: Get more finely tuned to your body, your feelings, and your Instrument Panel. For one week, notice throughout your day, "I feel this, I feel that." "This is what I feel right now." No faking. No judging. No trying to fix or change it—let it be what it is. You are where you are. Celebrate the feelings you love—accept the ones you don't like as temporary *and valuable*. Most people have gotten so used to negative emotion that they think it's normal and just sit in it unconsciously. Awareness is power. To get the big results, don't just read—practice! You're going to be thinking all day anyway, might as well use your thoughts deliberately. You'll be astonished at what happens over time.

APPLY IT USING YOUR WHOLE BODY: If you are more numb or often not sure what you feel, get your body into the act instead of doing this mentally. Get up and strike a pose for each feeling on the Instrument Panel from bottom to top, using your whole body. Act them out. Physical movement gets your cells and atoms moving too. Feel which feelings have slower or faster energy. Be silly toward the top.

Do these activities if you want to experience the results you've read about. Write in your journal how it felt. What did you notice?

Did you really get up and move? Before you read on, go back if you didn't!

Tip the Nose UP

JUST AS DOVES ARE THROWN ALOFT in happy celebration at weddings and ceremonies, Grace lifts you aloft as you practice Divine Openings. As you practice Divine Openings you'll be able to let in more and more of that Grace—the gift that cannot be "earned" by one's own efforts. Grace does 90% of it for you in the Non-Physical where the larger part of everything is created. I capitalize Non-Physical because to me it's another name for God.

Even after Grace lifts you and does 90% of it for you, you still need to do your 10%: point your beak where you want to go and flap your wings occasionally. Keep your beak tipped up, not aimed at the ground. The coming chapters are filled with wonderful, pleasurable ways to do your 10% to stay up there—it's not work: it's simply awakening, awareness, and allowing.

Grace has been raining on you all along, but if you can't let it in you can feel like you're dying of thirst even in a rainstorm. The Divine Openings in this book expand and open your pipes so you can allow in more Grace and ease. You will feel moments of causeless happiness or lightness.

After each burst of happiness or bliss, Law of Attraction might nudge you back down a bit, toward your old, established set point. Your set point is sticky, so it tends to pull you back down a bit after a big gain in altitude. Great good shines light into the shadows, and lights up the lower vibrations still lingering there. Softly accept what is revealed, and use the tools you're learning when that happens.

We find that people do not sink back into their previous lows again unless they resume seeking and reverse their progress, or get sloppy and don't do their 10%. It doesn't just happen by accident.

Law of Attraction is on your side once you've stabilized higher, though. It helps you stick at the new set point, and pulls you back up when you dip. Then you can gain more altitude and stabilize even higher, until you're flying high. Incremental rises are easiest to sustain. That's all you can do sometimes, and it's enough. If you judge it "not enough," that tips the nose down and altitude drops.

Appreciate every tiny tailwind, lift, and small gain. Appreciation always gains you extra altitude. More good things come your way. Just as appreciation accelerates your results—self-judgment and complaining reverses them. As you enjoy your way up, step-by-step, you'll stabilize so powerfully at each level that in the future, with a little attention to your Instrument Panel, you'll catch the slightest dip quickly and correct your course. Best of all, you'll get "rubberized"—you bounce off the bottom and snap back quickly. You can't be brought down for long.

A woman had come to me sad and clinically depressed, but for her second session she showed up much higher on the Instrument Panel. She complained, "Things got better, but now I'm frustrated and aggravated a lot." She was giving herself a hard time—thinking this aggravation was wrong. I suggested, "You came here depressed and in despair, at the bottom of the Instrument Panel. Where is aggravation on your Instrument Panel? Let's look."

"Wow, I'm way up there near the halfway mark already, after one session!"

"Yes, you have moved up from the bottom to the middle, and you are now pointed in an upward spiral. Stabilize there, just *enjoy being aggravated* for a while, and you'll move on up. We judge certain emotions as bad, and none of them are bad; they are *all good information*. Keep your nose tipped up and heading in a general upward direction toward more relief—that's all it takes. If you relax and allow yourself to feel what you authentically feel, Grace does the rest. Make it right, and experience that aggravation deliberately, powerfully."

Soften around the feeling and then point your nose upward.

Develop a habit to check your Instrument Panel routinely to see where you are, what your altitude is, and which way you're headed, just like a pilot does. The readings on your airplane's Instrument Panel are neither wrong nor right; they're information. Using your Instrument Panel, you can navigate anywhere. If you don't use it, you often end up in unexpected places, experiencing things you don't want, and wondering how you got there. The good news is: if you point your plane at San Francisco and keep the nose tipped up, not down, you *will arrive there.*

If I point the nose of my plane even slightly toward the ground, I will eventually intersect with the ground. If I point the nose of the plane level or upward, I will continue flying and reach my destination.

Don't confuse this with old-paradigm positive thinking—this is learning to navigate and plan your trajectory deliberately, and we'll add more such skills as we go. Your mind often resists positive thinking, arguing that it's "not true." Your mind will accept this.

One day I was happily writing, but as time to teach a class approached the nose tipped down as I thought about having to stop writing. I noticed the drop and adjusted my focus to how much fun it would be to start writing again after the class. I reminded myself how much fun classes are. Downward spirals start in such innocent ways, so take care to tip the nose back up.

If you are feeling good about a subject, and your nose is pointed up, you're going to like the manifestation you're cooking up. If you're feeling bad about a subject, and your nose is pointed down, you're probably not going to like the manifestation you're lining up. How valuable is it to be able to feel and forecast your results in advance? As you get more attuned to feeling, you'll have plenty of time to get in alignment with your Large Self and so achieve the outcome you want.

If you're in depression or frustration or at any lower altitude, now you know that to get back to being your Large Self you need to point the nose up and move up the Instrument Panel.

The game is to feel a little better. We've been told for so long that feeling bad is just the human condition; we believed we were supposed to gut it up and tolerate feeling bad. So we allowed ourselves to stay at low altitudes, not realizing how damaging that is over time. Even when something bad happens, feeling bad won't get you anything—even if everyone agrees how wronged you were. That victim feeling attracts more victimization. It's not worth the measly reward of being right. Take the controls, tip the nose up, and change your course now. Changing how you feel now changes your tomorrow. Notice and accept where you are, and then "intend" to climb.

Decades ago, in that recurring dream where I had my "control panel" in my hands, I felt powerful.

Upon awaking, I'd panic as it slipped out of my fingers and faded. Now I often have abstract dreams of esoteric knowledge that eludes me as I wake. It's exciting to wonder what new revelations will come out of those dreams in time. Notice that I'm not lamenting that I don't instantly know what each dream means—that would tip the nose down. I acknowledge that it does translate eventually—that tips the nose up. I'm playfully curious, and savoring the ongoing unfolding.

Make a lifelong decision that feeling a little bit better is the most important thing in the world.

SUMMARY: Unwanted or "negative" emotions are useful. They tell you where you are. You're supposed to feel bad when the nose of your plane is tipped even slightly downward, so you're alerted to the long-term consequences you're creating. A slight tipping up of the nose of your plane has enormous long range consequences, changing your trajectory, and eventually, your life.

It's not important to get to the highest altitude right away—just get the nose tipped up a bit. Get headed in the general direction you want to go. Just go for a little feeling of relief. You must value small gains—they mean everything in the long run.

Keep the nose of the plane tipped up.

Here's how to tip the nose up step-by-step:
Note where she is on the Altimeter (in bold) and how she moves up slowly and stabilizes at each point:

"I just feel **worthless** that Bill doesn't love me. I can't muster any energy to change my life. Wow, I'm low on the Instrument Panel. First I'll soften into that feeling of unworthiness and just breathe through it. Knowing where I am gives me direction. OK, where I am is where I am, so I'll be with this. I know what I want—to *feel better* about myself!"

"I'm **sad and depressed** because Bill doesn't love me. I can soften around this sad feeling and allow it to be for a bit, make room for it in my heart without trying to make it go away. Being sad feels bad—that's good because it's telling me I'm out of alignment with my Large Self"

"I'm **angry** about this powerlessness! I want my power back! What is he, stupid? Can't he see? Oh, that's good. I'm breathing and my energy is rising. Whew, I think I'll take a walk and soften into and allow this anger to move. I'll be here for myself and not talk to him or anyone about it. I hate this victim vibration!"

Next day: "I'm **discouraged,** but that's up the Instrument Panel from anger. Yes!!! Hmm, well at least I know I'm closer to the party! I'll take a break from relationships until I get clearer. I give up; it's too discouraging to keep trying because my old story about relationships is creating the same old outcome. I'm practicing a new way to be. Onward to the party!"

"I could try soothing myself before I talk to him, then I'll come from a place that's easier to hear. If I am easy on myself, that softening moves me up the Instrument Panel. Ahhh…I can do that."

"That feels better—not great, but better. Better is all I need for this moment."

"I am **confused** that I don't know what to do about this complicated situation. It's too **overwhelming** to try to talk to him just yet. Talking with him isn't helping."

"It's **frustrating** when I've tried so many things so many times. Ahh, I've been trying to manipulate him into loving me! I hate feeling frustrated, but I will allow this feeling and softly be with it!"

"Maybe I can just soften and **accept** how I feel about what he's up to, let go, and let God handle it. I'm **bored** with the whole thing—forget about him for a while. I'm going dancing."

The next week: "Ah, softening helped me let go! This feels **hopeful** at least. I don't have to figure it out, but I can daydream about the **possibilities**. If it's not him, then there's someone better for me, someone who naturally adores me. I feel *relief* right now. I'm above the Tipping Point! I'll do something fun while my Large Self handles it. I'll get a nudge if there's any action for me to take."

Whatever feels better to you is "up."

When you feel even slight relief, claim a victory. If you were out of shape and started training for a marathon, you would have to be happy with *small daily improvements* or you would never make it. Practice softening and allowing just to gain confidence that you can move, even if only slightly.

For now, forget changing your outer world. Focusing on that is so big it just gets you tense. Instead just do your 10%: your only job is to feel a tiny bit better each day and let Grace and momentum do the other 90%. Use your Free Will to witness, soften, and allow your feelings, and point the nose up when you can. Outer changes come naturally as you change inside. They have to—it is a Law of the Universe.

Raise your altitude *just because it feels better,* rather than because you want the guy, the girl, the job, the house, or the money. Do it for you. Do it because you've decided feeling as good as you can in this moment is your aim. Your life will always be *this moment,* and if you are a little bit happier in *this moment,* and this moment, and this moment, you change the entire trajectory of your life. You can't control outer circumstances, but you can *choose* how to *focus* in this moment.

Is the nose of my plane tipped up or down?

Getting out of pain and struggle is step one, and this book gets you there. Then there is no limit; you can create ever-increasing happiness and success. When you were young you felt the truth of the Instrument Panel. You knew how to move up it naturally. I am here to remind you of what you knew, before you were trained to ignore your own inner guidance. Master this and you are begin to live as your Large Self playing in material reality, consciously and joyfully—full out.

Soothe yourself that today's feelings create tomorrow's reality.

APPLY IT TO YOUR LIFE:

1. Fill your mind with uplifting input every day. Write in your journal any positive news, feelings, or steps you made, or miracles that happened that day. Briefly give your cares, worries, and missteps to The Presence. Let them go and don't retell the stories. *Don't listen to everything your mind says.*

2. Big successes are made of many small steps. Write a story that raises your altitude one small step at a time. Don't try to make too large a jump at one time. Don't get too hung up on "reality." There is no obligation to stick to the truth or be "accurate." *You* created *it*.

You soon begin to enjoy experiencing life softly, gently, with compassion for yourself. You stop complaining, analyzing, talking about it, or acting it out. When you need help, you talk to your Large Self more than other people. If you kept falling in a mud hole, you could wash yourself off every day, analyze with friends or a therapist how the hole got there and why you keep falling in, make it wrong that it's there—or you could fill in the hole, solving the root cause.

I'll remind you often, because when we experience an unwanted emotion or situation, the mind wants to make it wrong and spin us dizzy in the mental story. Our small self feels frantic to fix the situation. Address the vibrational root cause first and it's easier… or the problem entirely disappears.

Your vibration is the root cause.

Now, don't go digging for negativity—that creates years of futile, unnecessary processing. You actually create negativity and issues by looking for them and working on yourself, and it never ends (have you noticed that?) With Divine Openings, Life presents to you anything you need to deal with and you deal with it. Live life and be happy. Any feelings, events, or circumstances that need your attention will arise as needed in the course of normal living. Simple and elegant.

Let go of the old paradigm of clearing, healing, and learning lessons. "Working" on spiritual and personal growth is addictively ingrained into many well-meaning seekers. If you keep working on yourself, you'll be stuck on that hamster wheel forever. As soon as you decide your life is about pure evolution rather than "learning lessons" it gets really good. Evolution just *happens* with Divine Openings.

Anytime you feel something you don't like, life is telling you, "Here's a place where you're out of alignment with your Large Self, so it hurts." "Here's a place where you're not being your true self, so it's painful." "Here's an opportunity to raise your vibration, to feel better and evolve."

Get Yourself to the Party

WHEN YOU DESIRE something, your Large Self knows you want it, and instantly creates it in the Non-Physical. Snap! Done! Your Large Self starts that party for you right then and there. Ninety-nine percent of your desire is manifested and waiting for you—at the party. Where are *you?* Your job is this and only this: to get your vibration up to speed with the party, high on the Instrument Panel on that subject. You're the guest of honor, the party is poised at 99% complete, ready to begin. The hall is decorated, the band is tuning up, the food is on the table, and the guests are all standing there, waiting for *you*, the guest of honor. But this party can't start without *you*, because it's *your party*. Are you the missing element at your own party? Do you trip yourself up thinking of parties you didn't get to in the past, worry that there won't really be any party, that something will go wrong, or no one will come?

Soothe your mind's doubts, and focus with all your heart on getting to the party. Soften around the doubts, and allow them to be there. Talk about the party, ways to get there, and what you want rather than the doubts, and you'll get to the party *faster!* That last puzzle piece, that last 1% is your allowing the party to start in the physical. I want to make a T-shirt that says, "I *AM* the party!"

I'm not saying "never talk to anyone about your challenges," but do it sparingly, because *as you speak*, you focus energy, *thus you create*. Commiseration is *co-misery* that plummets your altitude. Speak your challenges quickly, and then shift to focus on the millions of *possibilities*.

I rarely speak of problems to friends. Why? Direct-to-The-Presence is the most powerful place to go with questions or challenges. Friendship is not about emotional support or problem-solving for me *at all* anymore. When I'm with friends and loved ones, it's all about living, loving, laughing, *and fun*.

Now you can navigate to the party!

You'll Feel It Before You See It

IT'S A GREAT COSMIC JOKE that what is most real is invisible and Non-Physical. Love, life force, compassion, magnetism, gravity, hope, and the intention and energy that precedes physical materialization are invisible, but very powerfully real. You can't always see, touch, hear, feel, or smell it. The physical "reality" we can see and touch is much less real and lasting—it's fleeting and impermanent.

As physicists know, things that seem to be solid really are not—they're mostly space. Your physical senses are now evolving to perceive a broader spectrum of reality. You'll begin to see, hear, know, and feel more that isn't yet physical. The more sensitive you become to Non-Physical pre-manifest energy, the more you can tangibly feel things long before they pop into the physical. Now the Non-Physical world is much more real to me than the physical world.

It's so helpful to feel yourself headed toward negative manifestations while you're still miles away– while you still have plenty of time to change your vibration and alter your course. When you feel bad, you'll be able to say, "Hmmm, I know this is not leading where I want to go, so how do I lift my altitude and adjust my course?" And you can enjoy the feeling of good things coming before they ever arrive!

You'll know what you're creating long before it materializes simply by noticing how you feel *about that subject*, instead of realizing afterward that your vibration *on that subject* had been low. You'll also get the bliss before the desired thing arrives—so you won't even be surprised when things you've wanted for years show up.

Again, there are no "bad" emotions or Instrument Panel readings. They're all indicators of alignment or misalignment with your Large Self on a particular subject. Emotions tell you where your nose is pointed, in case you hadn't noticed!

A "realist" friend and I are standing outside looking at the thirsty trees and grass, and I really want some rain. I'm surfing on a wave of happy anticipation of rain. Fifty miles to the east a great storm swells out of nowhere, and I smell it coming. The realist says, "We're in a drought. There's no rain in the forecast, I see no rain, and no rain's coming." The rain comes. Ah, the sweet scent of rain on dry grass.

The money, love, or experience you want is there, even if you can't see it. Get on and ride the wave of its coming. You can enjoy it now. It's real. It's right there in the Non-Physical.

What's most real is often invisible.

Sometimes I like to drive to the mountains. Three quarters of the way there, the flat road stretches out for fifty miles ahead without a hill in sight. It looks nothing like the vacation we're aiming for, but of course we don't turn around just because we don't see a single shred of evidence of mountains yet. The road signs say we're pointed in the right direction. We find ways to enjoy the drive—listen to music, laugh, anticipate, stop to take photographs or hikes.

We're nearly there and still all we see are a few small, unimpressive foothills. Compared to our visions of snow-capped mountains it's not very exciting—pretty un-spectacular. This would be a bad time to take score on whether we'll ever arrive. We keep driving. It's the very last fraction of the drive before we actually see mountains. Wow, there they are, their peaks slicing into the brilliant blue sky. The air gets chilly and crisp, the scent of pine fills the air, and a cold, clear stream winds alongside the highway. We see a lovely mountain cottage to stay in. It's been worth the drive. Now take score!

Your journey can be like that. No evidence, no evidence, no evidence . . . then, BOOM! Big evidence. It snowballs all along, but you don't see it until the snowball rolls up to you.

Keep going, and enjoy getting there. If you feel yourself flagging, losing hope, doubting, talk to yourself like you'd talk to any friend who was losing their direction: "It's waiting for me! I don't have to do everything—The Divine does the heavy lifting. As long as I don't turn back, I'll get there. All I have to do is keep the nose up, point in that general direction, keep moving, and I will arrive."

Take score only when the score is in your favor.

Self-Soothing

The Grace of Divine Openings soothes you, and I want you to learn to soothe yourself! It's a key skill—part of doing your 10%. Find a feeling of relief for yourself by choosing soothing words and tones of voice. Softly soothing yourself tips the nose upward.

How would you talk to a child or a friend in need? You wouldn't say, "Unimpressively slow progress! You'll never get there!" No, you'd say, "Oh, look, you're feeling just a little bit better! Good for you! Keep going!" Do that for yourself. To raise your altitude, talk soothingly to yourself until you feel a slight shift, not a dramatic shift. Just go for a little higher altitude. Step by step, and with the help of Grace, you can raise yourself to a very good place, and after wobbling a bit, stabilize eventually and stay up there.

I've never flown an airplane myself, but I've known enough pilots and watched enough movies to know that if you jerk the stick back and try to climb several thousand feet too quickly, you risk stalling, destabilizing your aircraft, and crashing. By the same analogy, a steady ascent is easier on you, your life, your family, and your body. Attempt to gain just a little altitude each day, each week, each month, and you will stabilize at each new altitude and maintain your gain permanently.

You've probably seen what happens when sudden fame strikes, and a person who is not accustomed to those heights can't maintain it, crashes, and melts down. Studies show that most people who win the lottery end up back where they started within a couple of years. The outer addition of money doesn't change their lives permanently, because they weren't vibrationally ready to maintain that altitude. It has been postulated that if all the money in the world were redistributed equally between everyone, within two years it would be back in the same hands it's in now. Law of Attraction supports that theory. With no change in vibration about money, most people would recreate their former state, for better or for worse. When you try to fly much, much higher than you're used to flying, it can be hard to stabilize. But when you rise gradually, Law of Attraction supports you and you stabilize at each new incremental level.

Contentment and boredom are actually nice resting places right above the Tipping Point. The release of tension that occurs at those points is a great relief. It's not bliss yet, but it's on the way there, and now momentum is on your side. Release resistance to where you are by softening and allowing where you are—that frees you to let momentum help you. If you're rising in altitude, and you feel like doing nothing, do nothing. Give the energy time to build. You're probably dog-tired from being in resistance for so long and need a break.

Practice choosing thoughts that tip the nose up and even slightly raise your altitude on every topic in your life until it becomes a natural habit. Write your rises in altitude and other successes in your journal until the resistant mind begins to get that *this is actually working*.

SUMMARY: Your job is to notice what you feel, witness it, and let Grace assist you. Just set the intention to tip the nose of your plane up.

What Stories? I Don't Hear Any Story!

STORIES RUN CONSTANTLY through our minds, and whether we're aware of them or not they shape our perception of the world, other people—and create our reality! Surely you've read this and maybe even studied it in depth, but have you really mastered it? Are subconscious stories still running your life? Many people who've been on the spiritual path for decades come to us, and they tell us with Divine Openings they finally "got it!"

As your awakening deepens with the assistance of Grace, you will master those tricksters we call stories. You'll notice whether a story is pointing your nose up or down.

It can take a little practice to learn to even recognize our "stories." Because stories run through your head constantly, twenty-four hours a day, even in sleep, you may not notice them at all. We're so accustomed to the mind's chatter that it operates outside awareness, like an underground aquifer. Before Divine Openings most of our stories were unconscious, but with your awakening you begin to witness them. This is vitally important because stories affect us whether we know they're running or not.

All our lives we've been telling ourselves stories, or being told stories, and believing them to be "facts." Stories are more fiction than fact—they're merely the mind's interpretations, dramatizations, distortions, analyses, and commentary. They are very rarely a pure, objective, factual description of a situation. Police reports are notoriously inaccurate—five people observing the same act will see five different things.

Notice whether a given story is beneficial to you. Deeply question its accuracy and always suspect your mind of bias. Focus on the stories that are helpful, and replace the ones that aren't before they hijack your energy.

Intend to hear yourself think and talk.

Some stories you tell other people, and some you tell to yourself. Be mindful of both, for they both create reality. For example, if you don't enjoy your job, you might say tell this unproductive story to yourself or another person as you drive to work: "Going to work is not fun. Why does it feel so bad? Hmmm, let's analyze where this feeling came from. It was my mother's domineering nature, etc., etc. … Should I quit? I shouldn't be feeling like this! I've been working on this issue for twenty years! When am I ever going to just get a great job and stop all this suffering? This job is holding me back. My co-workers are all so negative. But I can't quit because I'm afraid of having no money."

The pure fact is that *you have a low vibration feeling about your job.* Telling such a story to yourself or others, no matter how true you think it is, keeps the story spinning you in circles, and the reality doesn't change.

Stories gain momentum and spin into mental cyclones. The story and the emotion it magnifies spins up a reality you don't want. A story's spin generates a gravitational pull that attracts "like energy and circumstances"—evidence that the story is true. Evidence piles up and creates a belief, and that belief becomes an entrenched reality. *Your energy* is used to maintain those stories and beliefs.

It's all too easy to get caught up in a story "about" how wrong something was or is, why you're here, whose fault it is, and how powerless you are to change it. Those stories create you as a poor, good victim who has been wronged. "True" or not, it still leaves you a victim. The negative story is justified, fed energy, grows, and holds you in the drama like glue.

Stories justify and rationalize why it's true, or why you're right, but the price of that is high: it holds unwanted realities in place. You forget that you are the author of the story, or that you "bought the story" from someone, even someone who meant well. We inherit generational stories from our families.

It's all just information. Wherever you are is okay, because from this day forward, by looking at your Instrument Panel, you will know which way is up from where you are.

"Truth" is not the issue here. Where you are is "true" only because you created it, or you bought into a reality someone else created. You made it true. It's temporarily true till you create something else! You can now create something else you like better and make that "true." Changing your story about it helps you feel more powerful, and feeling powerful creates powerful realities.

SUMMARY: Every story spins up a vibrational vortex, which then attracts more people, things, events, and feelings like it. For better or worse, stories spin, generating the same feelings and manifestations over and over. If you listen to yourself think and talk you hear your stories. Never automatically accept what your mind says as true. All of it is story—some of it helps you, some of it doesn't. Witness your thinking, notice its effect on your vibration, and replace stories and thoughts if they are aiming you toward an unwanted reality.

Before you can fully master the powerful and revolutionary foundational methods of Divine Openings in the coming pages, you'll need to stop automatically believing your stories. This takes away their power to hijack your reality and rightfully restores that power to you.

Don't believe everything you think!

APPLY IT IN YOUR LIFE: Whenever you witness yourself indulging in a story, STOP and ask yourself: "Does this story make me feel *better,* or *worse?*" Practice talking to yourself in soothing tones, telling yourself a better "story" that even slightly tips up the nose. All you need is a few steps up the Instrument Panel to create upward momentum, and changes start to show up in your world.

It isn't always a negative story that holds you back. It can be a positive story that served you at one time, but now doesn't. One student owned a mid-sized computer business, and struggled with attracting good employees. He had all the clients he needed, but couldn't find enough qualified people to service them. At first we couldn't isolate the vibration preventing him from finding good people. I referred a brilliant unemployed technician friend to him, but interestingly, the technician kept finding excuses not to call him!

Then we realized the owner had started his business with the belief that there were too many inept technicians out there fixing computers, and that his mission was to be "the guy who did it right." This made him a successful sole proprietor, but held him back from expanding—his old belief that he was the only qualified person was now working against him. He kept attracting those inept technicians he had set out to save the world from, and repelled the good ones like my friend who didn't match his story. He let it go and competent technicians started applying.

Our stories play out in our reality—and so create our reality.

Another student's esteemed mentor had told him, "never pay for work you could do yourself." This was great when he had a whole karate school full of volunteer labor, but later, in another business, being the Lone Ranger exhausted him and nearly put him out of business. One day he realized that story had to go so he could hire help.

Whether a story is "true" or not is a tricky and irrelevant distraction. The important question to ask about any story or thought are, "Does it make me feel better, or worse?" "Is it limiting, or empowering?"

How does telling this story make me feel?
What reality is it creating?

Live Your Life, Not Your Stories

THE ULTIMATE REWARD of becoming aware of your stories is simple, but profound and beautiful: one day the mists part and you find yourself experiencing Life directly, purely and simply like a child, without the distortions and complicated mental commentary *about it.* The mind is blissfully quiet.

When you're making love, you're experiencing it, not thinking about it. When you're working, you're immersed in the task, with no tortuous story running about how hard it is. When you're sitting outside, you're alive with the pleasure of breathing, air on your skin, sounds caressing you ears. When you're doing a task you've done a thousand times, it is the first time. There's no story about how it should be, or used to be, or might be someday. You're having an experience in this moment.

Increasingly you're living life without so many filters, distortions, stories, beliefs, and faulty interpretations. You're responding fresh in the moment—not reacting from old beliefs, habits, and patterns, all of which are hardened, fossilized stories. You're spontaneous, innocent, and flexible, not a pre-programmed robot doing what you've always done and thinking what you've always thought. Life is wondrous when you experience each sparkling new moment uniquely as it is rather than through the dirty windows of a tired old story.

We dive deep into that blissful, no-story, No-Mind state in the 5-Day Retreats. Together we enter the profound peace and bliss of a quiet, still mind with no stories—in the exponentially amplified energy field of the group. Once you've experienced that pristine state, it's easier to find it again and again. You know the address of Grace.

The Divine Opening below expands your consciousness so that you can witness yourself more clearly. It also prepares you to receive one of the most powerful Divine Openings practices: Diving In.

SUMMARY: We need stories and thoughts to comprehend and navigate a linear life—but witness your stories mindfully—for they shape your reality. Create your stories deliberately so you're supported, not limited by them. Life becomes fresh, new, innocent, and magical when you *experience your Life instead of your stories.*

Divine Opening

LOLA INVOKES a powerful Divine Mother vibration here.
You can enjoy as many of this Divine Mother Hug type of Divine Opening as you like, as often as you like, because they do not accelerate your energy and do not require assimilation time. They are soothing, calming, and grounding. Gaze, then close your eyes and relax.

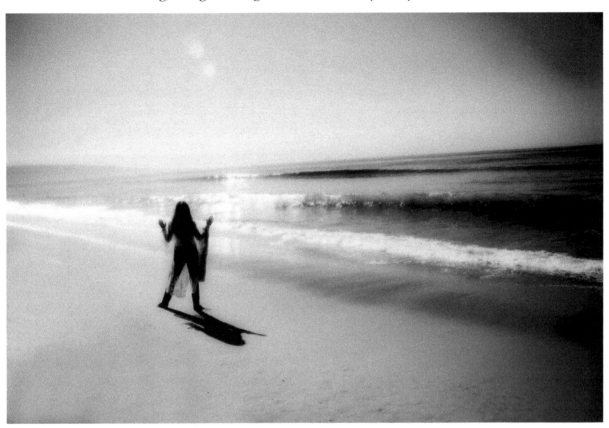

Figure 2—Lola Jones by the sea. Photograph by Carola Gracen.

Diving In, a Life-Changing Foundational Practice

I DEVELOPED THIS DIVING IN METHOD to help you gain the same freedom from lower emotions, suffering, and struggle that I experienced in my twenty-one days of solitude and silence. Tipping the nose up and Diving In both lead to feeling good, but are used in different situations. Tipping the nose up is routine mental maintenance—Diving In is deep and life-altering on a broad scale.

Tipping the nose up is for managing the mind's random thoughts that offer themselves to you as you go through your daily life, because those thoughts create vibrations that then create reality. Diving In is amazingly effective for long-standing, old, strong or recurring feelings, beliefs, or patterns—for reclaiming masses of tied up power.

If tipping the nose up fails or the feeling returns, it's time to Dive In.

Diving In gathers similar vibrations together and raises them en masse, very often permanently., sparing you from years of processing individual issues one by one. Decades of stubborn issues melt into allowing and acceptance, restoring lightness and freedom to your entire being. Receiving Divine Openings also loosens the backlog of stagnant energy, helping it rise.

More importantly, Diving In soon frees you from *resistance to feeling* in general. The end goal of Diving In *isn't to make feelings go away*. It's to accept all feelings. You return to that natural childlike state when you felt feelings in the moment, and they simply moved. Children and animals immediately feel every feeling, the vibration moves up, and they move on. You will return to living in the moment, as you are designed to do. When you reach enlightened equanimity, you will feel all feelings but not linger in them or suffer over them. You'll allow and value all feelings, and you'll bounce back up easily. You'll develop extraordinary resilience.

When you resist an emotion, it drops down in vibration even more, and gets tucked away in your body and energy field—it doesn't go away. If you've *"spiritual bypassed it"* or ignored it, it still vibrates in you and attracts things like it. When you softly Dive In, accept, and feel, it quickly passes. It's so simple you will soon wonder why you didn't think of it all along. Therapists, Divine Openings Guides, and Divine Openings students rave about how fast it works.

How to Dive In and Drop the Story

THE KEY TO DIVING IN is to dive into the feeling and drop the story (the talk, the words.) The story is the smoke, just a symptom—the feeling is the fire, the real cause. The feeling is where you'll find relief and reclaim your long-lost power. You wouldn't try to put out a fire by blowing the smoke away. Just as blowing the smoke fans the fire and makes it grow, when you tell a problem story or talk about a problem too much, it fans the fire but never, ever puts it out.

The story is a valuable fire alarm *alerting you to the feeling*, so appreciate that briefly, and then drop the story and give your complete, compassionate attention to the feeling, the vibration. The distracting, spinning, inflammatory story's job is done once it has pointed you to the feeling.

The story is a self-perpetuating distraction. The feeling is where the power is.

Magic happens when you tend to your feeling/vibration first rather than leap into using words or actions to fix the situation. Always begin by allowing and accepting your *own* feelings *about the situation*. It doesn't mean you have to like the feelings, or the circumstance that sparked the feeling, it means you *allow and accept the feeling so it can move.*

It is what it is, so you might as well choose to *accept what is* in this moment. Resistance is like glue holding you to what you don't like. Let's do what works: lower vibration moves up more easily with acceptance of the feeling. Acceptance is a vibration just above the Tipping Point in the middle of the Instrument Panel—then upward momentum kicks in.

The story generates endless loops of the unwanted feeling until it's a spinning cyclone of negative energy—it makes you feel worse, more stuck, and it never resolves. With this powerful Diving In process, you'll *never dive into the story*. You'll witness and acknowledge the story, then drop it, and *feel the feeling itself, in your body,* with no words, no story.

How to tell when you've dropped the story? There are <u>no words</u> in your head.

This powerful step-by-step Diving In process raises even persistent, life-long, core, lower feelings en masse, because it attracts other vibrational threads like it and raises all of them at once, resulting in profound feelings of peace, and sometimes euphoric release. No more endless issue-by-issue processing.

Every time you feel a feeling you don't like, don't analyze: practice this core Diving In process.

- Sit, close your eyes, and notice the story about that area of your life. Let the story and the characters in it become a rope that you can follow down out of your head and into the feeling in your body. Drop down into the pure feeling sensations.

- Give all your attention to the *feeling in your body* that's underneath the story. Imagine diving into it, and *soften and embrace it* like an old friend (which it is.)

- Breathe gently into it, like a baby breathes. Let your spine undulate gently. Breathe *softly* into the feelings and sensations; be kind to yourself.

- Name the sensations if you wish: tight, achy, numb, warm, itchy, heavy, stabbing pain, etc.

- Say "yes" quietly to the *feeling sensation*. This helps you *soften and allow it to be.* "I hate this feeling, but it's here, so I will soften around it. Power is tied up in it, and I want my power back."

- The moment you softened and *accepted the feeling itself* you are already above the Tipping Point on the Instrument Panel on that subject. Wow, you have raised your vibration, and momentum will help you rise more.

- To try a bit more advanced version: experience the feeling as just atoms vibrating in your body. It is just a vibration!

- A little relief is enough—remember, momentum will carry you upward. Open your eyes, notice how you feel.

APPLY IT TO YOUR LIFE: Stop reading now. Get still and slow your breathing down. Get some paper. People often tell us they didn't truly reap the big magic of Divine Openings until they practiced it mindfully in their lives, and in these experiential activities, so let's Dive In right now! For your first practice, choose a small to medium subject, not a huge issue. Choose a drama, situation, story, or feeling you'd like to be free of. Write just a couple of sentences of the story to help you tap into the feeling. You don't even need a name for the feeling, just feel it. Now tear out and crumple up the page, drop the story, and focus 100% on the feeling and how it feels in your body. Use the Diving In process above to get to acceptance. That's all you need for now.

Fortunately, now you won't often fall for those tricky stories that hijack your emotions before you know it. Whenever a person or situation is not pleasing to you, before speaking or taking action, inside your own mind and body, with eyes open, first briefly Dive In to *your own emotional response to it*. You'll be astonished how this simple habit transforms you, and then changes your reality.

The analogy of diving into the feeling as if it's a big pool of water deep in your body makes it easier for some. The air above is the surface story. Underwater you can't hear a story.

Raise your altitude slowly, step by step. Softening, acceptance, and a few steps upward are all you need at any one time. As you practice this *softening and allowing* while living your daily life, it becomes your new habit. Soon you notice a dramatic improvement in your ability to stay in the flow and be happy, and then to manifest and influence your world. People and circumstances seem to morph for you. It all begins with Diving In.

Mastery of Diving In brings rapid life progress, and because some people learn better and faster from audio and video guided meditations than from reading, we created a whole audio series to support you in mastering it, with more than 20 audios and videos to walk you through the Diving In process so you can relax and not have to think. If you feel that would serve you see Talk Audios in the site menu.

Practice Diving In it until it's your new automatic response to any story, issue, problem, or lower vibration. Practice until you can catch a story before it gets revved up and hijacks you. Even after you've been happy for years, sailing along on a steady high, if your vibration plummets, the *first* reaction of the mind will probably be to make it W-R-O-N-G. The *story* is, "I should be beyond this now. I shouldn't feel this way." Making it wrong adds resistance and prolongs your pain. As soon as you can gather your wits, soften, allow it, Dive In, value the message of those feelings, and let it rise to acceptance.

A couple of times I've said to myself out loud, "Pull it together, Lola. Dive In and drop the story. It will rise." And it does every time! If you try to make the feeling go away, have someone "heal" it or fix it, or talk about it and spin in the story, an opportunity to reclaim tied up power is lost. It's supposed to feel "bad" to be in a limiting story! "Bad" feelings point the way to a whole new freedom if you Dive In and free that tied up energy. You may need to Dive In more than once on the same subject, but with soft allowing, you'll get it.

You don't need to "heal" feelings—they're not sick—they're valuable vibrational indicators. If you feel anger at your mate, but try to fix her, or ignore the feeling, or rise above it, that vibration still hums away in you, attracting anger from your mate, bad drivers on the road, or maybe a stubbed toe. When you make the feeling wrong or push it away, you create resistance in your body. Over time, you get might progressively stronger signals like physical tension, pain, or things go wrong. A dis-ease or some unwanted event could manifest to get your attention if you ignore it too long.

If you try to fix something by analyzing the story, you're rearranging deck chairs on the Titanic to try to keep it from sinking. The hole in the boat was the root cause. Your feeling vibration is the root cause, and the story is a tricky distraction. Always go to the root cause—Dive In.

Some spiritual people try to do what I dubbed the "spiritual bypass." They try to go from the lower vibrations straight up to love and bliss. They'll tell me, "I try to surround the person I'm angry at with love and light, but it's not working." The feeling needs to be felt, allowed, and moved. Softly accept *your feeling about it*—then it can move. Once you drop the story, the Diving In process will get the energy moving upward, energy is reclaimed, and relief is found.

Pain and peace, bliss and anger are all made of Divine energy, but at different vibrational frequencies. Peace and bliss are freely flowing energy—their vibration is high and strong. Pain, fear, and anger are lower, slower, denser energies. Resisting emotions that feel bad only makes them slower, lower, and denser.

Energy alignment before action.

Your happiness is precious. Don't suffer! If you struggle with any aspect of Diving In, and need more intense and personalized support and guidance, refer to the resources in the back of the book.

Once you learn Diving In, use this short version:

- Drop the story, drop down into your body, and feel the feeling and the physical sensations.

- Breathe softly like a baby into the feeling. Embrace and allow it with compassion.

- Then feel it as vibrations only. Breathe for pleasure while you softly be with it, accept and allow it, in no rush for it to pass. Acceptance automatically puts you above the Tipping Point! This can take only minutes with some practice!

Drop the story. Feel the feeling in your body.

Even when you know this effective strategy for finding relief right in the middle of confusion or crisis one of the hardest things, when your thinking has been hijacked, is to *notice you're in a story*, remember to drop it, and Dive In to the feeling and vibration.

If you feel numb, Dive In to the numbness, and that too will move and resolve. Although most times you can Dive In and move a feeling quickly, there are times when you need to give yourself a day or two or even longer to be with it. If you Dive In and it doesn't move, go about your life, *letting yourself feel however you feel for a while.*

Everything is vibration—atoms moving around. Breaking it down into pure and simple vibration, your experience of the feeling without the story might go like this: "This is a feeling/vibration in my body," or "It's just atoms quivering. I can allow and be with that." You'll soothe yourself, "Everything vibrates. Notice how this vibration feels. Vibration *wants* to rise."

Emotion creates a physical vibration, and by diving into it and experiencing it without the story, you can let it move into a higher vibration. Pretty simple.

No story, no resistance = no suffering.

APPLY IT: Experience everything as vibration in your body this week, without story. Feel everything as atoms vibrating in your body, with no story labelling it "good" or "bad," no names for feelings, and no words about *why you feel that way*. Simply experience everything directly.

You'll get freer, happier, and even more intuitive and energy sensitive. Vibration is pre-feeling—you can feel it before there is even a feeling about it, long before it manifests as physical reality!

Diving gently into the feeling brings the power of your Divine Presence to the situation, lighting up new circuits, illuminating new choices. As you tune up your vibration, you'll be more clear-minded and aligned with your powerful Large Self. Then if there is still any problem left, you'll let go and let The Divine do the heavy lifting, or you'll be guided what to do. Everything moves and resolved more easily once there's no sticky negative emotional charge on it.

Any feeling un-resisted moves, rises, and frees you.

As you dive into a feeling, *"being with what is"* instead of resisting what is, energy flow is restored, relief is instant, and you are opened to even more good things to come. Even if it's only a little relief, you know the nose of the plane is tipped up a bit, which changes your entire trajectory. If you are flying along with the nose even slightly tipped down, you'll eventually hit the ground, but tipping up even slightly changes everything—*you won't hit the ground!* That makes all the difference in the world, and your future is altered.

You may in ten minutes raise abject fear or deep grief into bliss. With no story to keep regenerating the lower feeling-vibration, the pipes are opened, and more love and bliss flow through you.

An attorney, came to me with a lot of issues: a million dollar lawsuit against him, two runaway teen boys, a recent divorce, and his business going south. Within an hour he was feeling better, and in two sessions he was feeling better than he had felt in years, although nothing had materially changed yet. He looked stunned, but felt better. It radically disrupted his reality.

We believe change takes hard work and a long time. The mind thinks happiness is dependent on outer circumstances. Hey, anyone could be happy if everything and everyone around them was always agreeable. Mastery is choosing happiness independent of outer circumstances. He began an upward spiral after that, and his life opened up steadily. Three years later he was living his dream of working in the music business, putting on rock concerts. His most recent show starred—guess who? His two now prodigal sons.

The feelings that create the most problematic realities are the ones we've resisted the longest. If every feeling was a fresh, new, "now" feeling, it would not hook you or cause such a problem; it would flow on through you and upward, as feelings are designed to do. When it sticks with you and won't move up, or if it recurs frequently, you know you have a long-practiced habit of resisting feeling. There is a deep pool of similar unmoved vibration within you. A current situation can activate that old, well-practiced vibrational habit and make it seem as if all of that negative feeling is present right now, when in reality the bulk of it is a blast from the past. It blows a current problem out of proportion and hijacks your mind and emotions.

Remember this when you feel a really big charge on something: it's not about what's happening today, it's mostly old energy. Dive In, let Divine Grace assist you, and you not only get relief from the current situation, you recover that entire, enormous pool of energy. When you can softly be with the feeling and let it move, you are free, and back in the present moment with a clean slate. You're restored to your power as your altitude rises to the level where your Universal Source lives, which it naturally does when we soften. It's only our tensing up that stops energy flow, keeps our vibration low, and creates distress. When we allow the feeling to flow, we return naturally to wellbeing every single time.

It's often said that public speaking and heights are people's two greatest fears. From my experience with thousands of people, I'd put fear of feeling atop the list.

When you fear no emotion, you are free.

Be patient with yourself if you have many years of practice resisting, tightening up, and believing your stories. As you practice staying out of the story and softly accepting the feeling in your body, your vibrational setpoint goes higher with each success.

You'll catch yourself in a story and ask yourself, "Hmm, is this story productive? How does this story make me feel? Where does it take me on the Instrument Panel? This story is a trap! I'll feel this fully, and it will move upward naturally." After the charge is neutralized, you'll naturally create better stories to replace the disempowering ones.

Give yourself appreciation each time you catch a story, Dive In, and find even a little relief. Now you know that what you focus on consistently over time, you create more of, so focus on your successes. Don't let your mind dwell on what's still "wrong" or unresolved. Confidence builds, velocity increases. You'll prove to yourself that Diving In does work.

Whatever is holding you back, go to the root cause. For example, finding a mate: your scary or limiting stories can point you to the feeling underneath, for example: *"fear of being alone"* or the *"fear of being unlovable."* But then drop the story. Find a place of soft acceptance of the feeling—that is the essence of Diving In. New solutions open up when energy that was tied up in that feeling rises up the Instrument Panel.

It's the same with money difficulties. Forget money itself—it's just a byproduct of the root cause: your money vibration, your deep feelings about money. If thinking about money tightens you up, obviously, thinking about it doesn't help anyway. Dive into the *fear, unworthiness, or worry about money* deep in your body. Be with the feeling softly, not trying to change it, allowing it without running away. That energy begins to move, to rise in frequency, up the Instrument Panel. Go for feeling better at first, rather than increased money.

Note that when you judge the prosperous, you push money *away from you* at a vibrational level. Religions have for eons told us money and prosperity are evil, yet they have to use money to operate, too.

Check inside: how do you feel about money and people who allow in money? Dive into that *feeling*, drop the story, and as vibration rises, that judgment dissolves, allowing more money to come to you and stay.

Money is merely a form of appreciation you can exchange for value. It has no inherent quality of good or evil other than whatever story you bought from society or created about it. Your story creates your money reality. You need money to enjoy freedom and choice in your life. Organizations need money to pay their expenses and keep their dedicated people, and to reward those who create value. Celebrate and appreciate those who let in money, and you will allow in more too.

What you resist persists.

Pain + resistance = suffering.

Don't resist your resistance! Soften!

Now you know that feeling good is the most important thing in the world. When you're feeling good, your pipes are open, you're one with your Large Self, and Divine energy is flowing through you freely. Unwanted emotions and manifestations tell you you're vibrating lower than your Large Self on that subject. It's supposed to feel bad when your pipes are constricted. *Be glad* it feels bad to be your small self. Low vibration reminds you to let go, tip the nose up, or Dive In, and get back to where your Large Self is: always right there at home frequency.

To prove to you that Diving In is not about fixing anything or working on yourself, but truly a raising of vibration, try this: if you are already high on the Instrument Panel, Dive In to a good feeling, and it too rises. You go even higher. Dive In for pure fun. Your creativity flowers, and your passion soars to new heights. You find new levels of love.

While for most, Divine Openings brings an easy, sweet return to bliss, some of you believe nothing good comes without paying a price of pain. Some need to feel something intense and dramatic to know it's "working," and that belief in suffering will play out! Intend now to allow all feelings with acceptance, and let it be easier, and you'll be surprised to find things seem to have changed "for no apparent reason."

Remember, when you do feel strong lower vibrations moving, it can feel overwhelming for short periods, but that passes when you soothe yourself that it is very, very old energy. It is not happening now!

The days of trudging through emotions and issues for years are over. Now, once you Dive In and experience just a few deep, old emotions fully until they rise into acceptance or even bliss, you are on the way to being free from suffering and bondage to *all emotions forever.* You still have the entire range of emotions, but they don't run you.

The natural outcome of practicing the Diving In process is at some point, you seldom need to do it *formally* anymore. Feelings flow easily and naturally as they are supposed to do. You live Life instead of stories. You stop resisting feeling entirely. Lower feelings move, then you feel better. Health, well-being, and prosperity are all about raising vibration. When you flow emotional energy, money, relationship, creativity, fulfillment all open up. With acceptance, vibration automatically rises. Hurt, anger, and fear, after being experienced, rise to peace and bliss. New things begins to manifest around you.

You are on your way to bliss and peace and you never have to go back unless you get sloppy with your Free Will choices. Grace does 90% of the work. Do your small 10%..

The two main ways to handle a lower vibration:

1. Tip the nose up. Tell yourself a better story and move up the Instrument Panel.

2. If that doesn't work, or doesn't last, it's a sign to go deeper. **Dive In**, drop the story, and feel the feeling.

Should I Dive In, or Tip Up The Nose of the Plane?

A STUDENT ASKED, "How do you know when to Dive into the emotion and experience it fully so that it rises, and when to just tip the nose up and change your thoughts?" Both end up with you feeling better. Both have you value all feelings as messengers. Both teach you to let emotion and energy move freely.

Here is a helpful distinction: if you've tried repeatedly to raise your altitude on a particular subject by tipping the nose up, and it doesn't stay up, *Dive In*. There is probably a large stagnant pool of old, resisted feeling, a blind spot, a strongly practiced vibrational habit, or perhaps unconscious numbness. Most of us have vibrational habits we don't know we have. We've all picked up stories, habits of thinking, and beliefs by attuning to the energy of parents, teachers, society and others. Now it's on autopilot, and goes unnoticed. A feeling will come back even after Diving In if you resume telling the old story and create it again. Get the Diving In Audio/Video Set and take a webinar if you need help. Sometimes you just need an expert guide until you can fully be there for yourself.

If I feel anything less than good, I know that the small self has latched onto something contrary to what my Large Self feels. There's nothing to "do" except Dive In and feel. When I can just be there for myself, feel, and let it move up—it's that easy. Only when I resist is it harder.

I am where I am, and compassion and acceptance of that reduces resistance, and relieves me of the need to work on myself anymore. As enlightenment unfolds, the small self might find sneaky, subtle ways to keep us in stress. Many months after my twenty-one days of silence I built up some physical tension again, and asked The Indweller for insight.

Soon I had a dream in which I had been on a nice vacation and it was time to go home. I had left my baggage at the home airport on the way there. I had not missed it at all, but suddenly wanted it back when it was time to go home. I called to arrange the proper procedure to get my baggage back, and was suddenly feeling stressed. The feeling, tone, or vibration of a dream tells you more than the story line. My small self was saying, "OK, vacation over. I want the old familiar life back again." It didn't care that the old familiar life was way less fulfilling and wonderful. I woke laughing, knowing that my small self was trying to get back to familiar territory. I had even started drinking caffeine again, which makes me tense. I don't need caffeine to be energized, so why was I using it again? I stopped. Relaxation returned.

Your dreams may change dramatically with Divine Openings. We used to think we had to interpret or understand our dreams, but Divine Openings has taken the work out of that too. With Divine Openings, dreams don't require analysis—even "bad" dreams are nothing to worry about—the dream is moving the energy for you. Just *feel the dream*, notice your intuitions, if any, and take any action you're guided to. The rules change at different levels of consciousness.

You get benefits whether you remember the dream or not. Much of the "work" in Divine Openings is done in your dreams or in sleep when you're out the way entirely, and least resistant. Let it be that easy.

You may be kept awake in strange empty states. Just lie there, relax, breathe, snuggle yourself, and savor. Don't resist being awake and you'll get up rested. Normal "insomnia" is tension and resistance, but Divine Openings sleeplessness isn't insomnia—you could sleep only a couple of hours and still glow with boundless energy. I've laid awake all night receiving a download for a retreat or a project and felt wonderful all day the next day. Soften around it. Snuggle in. Let it be.

It's an Inside Job

PEOPLE TOO OFTEN try to fix what's making them feel bad by trying to change something or someone "out there." They think that if someone else changes their behavior, if they can talk it out, manipulate the circumstances, change jobs, make the world change—they will be happy. But if the world has to change before you can be happy, you're in big, big trouble! There are too many people and too many things that would have to change, and have you ever managed to change even *one* person? Does your government have to change before you can be happy? Does your body have to change first? Does your income have to change first? That's a tough way to go.

Your entire world shifts when you shift. No more working hard at challenges and trying to control people and circumstances. Change your altitude first. Hold off on actions and big decisions until you are high and clear. If you act when your altitude is low, you'll work too hard or create the same old things.

Now that you're learning to free tied up energy, you can use that power to create in the Non-Physical. You'll be amazed at the clarity, energy, and synchronicities that magically appear as you progress through this book—without working on yourself! You'll create with intention and vibration first. Then take action as guided. Guided actions are exponentially more effective.

You can cut your action to a fraction.

Life Begins to Flow

You're being prepared to go higher with the upcoming Divine Openings. Go slowly! If you feel an urge to skip ahead or rush, that's your mind's restlessness. *Slow down to build a solid foundation.*

Relief comes when you soften around "what is" first. You shift the energy before taking action or trying to fix it. When we fly into action too fast we work too hard trying to fix a situation without addressing its root cause: the vibration that's creating it. A low feeling might arise about work, relationship, or health. You stay out of the story—the mental talk in your head about it, and instead you allow the pure feeling. Something makes you sad, so you softly experience and allow the sadness without telling the story of why you're sad. You get fearful, so you feel the fear without telling yourself scary stories. Those feelings rise in vibration, and you feel relief. Best of all, you stop attracting those same old unwanted things to you.

You will at times find yourself tempted to run the story over and over in your head, analyze it, or tell it to others. Now you know that spins you in the drama, and can get you feeling like a victim or a righteous judge making the situation or person wrong. You know the story perpetuates that bad feeling and generates more of it, spinning the story larger, making the situation worse, plus attracting similar incidents. Develop the habit of recognizing the story, and accept what is in the moment so it can move. As enlightenment unfolds, you value being happy and loving more than being right about your story, and you choose to drop disempowering or upsetting stories.

What Happens as Your Vibration Rises

ONCE YOU CAN experience your emotions internally instead of playing them out externally, your life becomes a drama-free zone. I think back on times when I tried to stay out of conflicts and could not do it. Now it seems inconceivable to live in that kind of drama, and I laugh to myself, "What was I thinking?" But that was a different consciousness, and in this new consciousness, you'll find that so many of the old problems just don't exist anymore—it even seems odd that you ever had them.

Most conflicts and unhappiness with other people diminish once you realize how you created your part of those relationships. People begin to behave completely differently with you as you align with your Larger Self.

Typically the changes that happen as you raise your vibration fall into three categories:

1.) Other people shift in how they behave with you, circumstances morph.
2.) Your perception shifts and you're no longer bothered by what used to bother you.
3.) You part easily with who and what doesn't work for you, or it departs from your life.

Your greatest power is in raising your own vibration before speaking or acting on it. Many processes in the book help you master this. For now, try to make important decisions or key conversations when your vibration is high. Even if it seems like you must act right now, or fix something, you can almost always wait until you're feeling better unless the house is on fire. It may look like the cause of the emotion is "out there," but stay focused within, on your feeling response to the situation, where your power is. This becomes an empowering new habit.

Once you've experienced an emotion fully and reclaimed that tied up emotional energy, you have a clearer, wiser view of the situation, and your actions will be Grace-assisted, in the flow, and more effective. If you still need to say something to the other person after you've dealt with yourself, your words are cleaner and more effective. They can hear you, perhaps for the first time, and your relationship transforms in a lovely, easy way.

Lower vibrational feelings are usually for "internal use only."

Once you're clear, you speak from your Large Self with no emotional charge, and that attracts less emotional charge from others. From a powerful and pure place, you can tell someone how you feel or felt, or what you want, with no trace of victim energy. When "you are there for yourself" emotionally and energetically, others are more likely to be there for you. If you do blow up and vent on someone, you are human. Just take responsibility, clean it up, tell them you should have taken it within first, and you are back in integrity. They will respect you for that.

Once a relative criticized me in front of a friend, telling him all of my faults from her perspective. After going to bed, I dived in and felt through it, softening, allowing, and accepting without trying to fix it mentally. The next morning I was centered and in my heart, and I knew I could communicate well. When my friend left the room, I gave the relative a hug, and tears came to my eyes—not the tears of a victim or a blamer, but of an open heart. I spoke about "how I felt" rather than "what she did." I said, "It hurt when you said that about me, especially to him." She immediately apologized and I just listened as she talked about her unhappiness. She was very depressed about her husband's disability. Our relationship moved up to a new level.

There are times when you will use raw anger constructively to make a difference, to move yourself up from depression, fear, grief or despair, stand up to someone, help someone you love, or change a situation. Anger is powerful when used consciously—when you are its master rather than taken over by it unconsciously. Seize every opportunity to practice what you're reading in the real world. Any failure is just feedback for you. Keep practicing.

Why there is so much emphasis on emotion in Divine Openings:

- *Learning to manage your vibration helps you navigate through life* more successfully. Emotions are your Instrument Panel indicator of your vibration.

- *Once you master emotion you can manifest powerfully.* Experiences, bodily conditions, finances and relationships all reflect the emotional energy you're vibrating and radiating. When you can move emotional energy, you can move any energy. Manifesting is literally the ability to focus and flow energy.

- *Emotional mastery helps you sustain enlightenment.* No amount of esoteric knowledge can substitute for emotional mastery. It's possible to have flashes of profound illumination *but lose it* when confronted with emotional or challenging life situations. Paradoxically, when you can be with any feeling, you will feel good more of the time, and that helps sustain your enlightenment. Many people develop high spiritual knowledge, but their practical life still doesn't work well, or manifesting is hard. Emotional mastery opens up more success in every area of practical life.

Grace Supersedes Law of Attraction

THE BEST NEWS OF ALL is that Grace supersedes Law of Attraction, so you get free boosts to get you going, rather than having to ratchet your vibration up all on your own. Divine Openings is not a "do it all yourself" program like Law of Attraction, although we use the Law of Attraction. With Divine Openings, the Divine does the heavy lifting. Grace does 90%. Your job, your 10% is to train yourself to use your Free Will effectively to manage your vibration and to *go with the flow of that Grace.*

Law of Attraction does attract feelings, people, things, and experiences to match what you are already vibrating. If you're feeling bliss, Law of Attraction brings you more blissful feelings, people, things, and events. The Instrument Panel helps you pinpoint where you are on a particular subject, understand what you're attracting, and shift your vibration.

Like the laws of physics, Law of Attraction isn't personal. If Hitler and Gandhi both stood on a cliff and leaned forward, they would both fall and hit the ground. Gravity isn't personal, nor does it judge good or bad. Law of Attraction will help you stay high if you are high, but it will also contribute to keeping you at a low point if you are low. It has a "sticky" effect that pulls you back to the altitude that was your set point until you firmly claim a higher set point.

Like attracts like.

Law of Attraction and the Instrument Panel are not about how good or bad you are—they're about your alignment with your Large Self. You're not "bad" for being out of alignment with your Large Self—it just doesn't feel good or work in your favor. Allow compassion for where you are. Soften up on yourself and you instantly move up to the acceptance point, pretty high on the Instrument Panel. Appreciate that elevation and you get another one. Say to yourself, "I'm glad it doesn't feel good to be out of alignment with my Large Self!" You'll get another instant elevation.

You're not "bad" at a low altitude—you're just pointed at destinations you won't like. You're not "good" because you're at a high altitude—but when you're up there in alignment with your Large Self you're headed someplace that you'll like.

From depression, fear, sadness or despair, your inborn instincts know (or used to know) that anger is a powerful move upward. You were born with an instinct to get angry to get your power back when you get scared, sad, or depressed. As a child you knew anger felt better, more powerful than despair. But what were we told as children when we got angry? "You're being bad!" "Be nice." "You're going to get a spanking!" We'd get angry, get bad reactions from people, and then stuff it and go back down to depression; then our natural instincts to get angry would kick back in and we'd get angry, then someone would say we shouldn't do that. We'd ping-pong: anger, depression, anger, depression—or anger, fear, anger, fear—so we'd never make it all the way up the Altimeter. Some of us lost our Instrument Panel, turned it off, or got it turned upside down.

Let yourself use the bridge of anger, and you can ease up to frustration. From there you can rise above the Tipping Point to acceptance, boredom, peace, or hope, where momentum increases automatically. Soon you're flying high as your Large Self.

When you're feeling anger, revenge and blame, if you talk to friends who just take your side and support your "story," that won't help at all. Take it to The Presence. Your anger will soon pass, leaving you with more productive feelings. When we speak angry feelings to another person it can escalate, and if they don't know how to raise their vibration they may have a hard time letting it go later, even though you've moved up the Instrument Panel and feel great. Raise your altitude first, and then speak to them from your Large Self; if you have something tough to say you'll say it more effectively. Your Large Self can say tough things with compassion. I've even had people thank me later for getting mad at them!

People want us to do what feels good to them, not what feels good to us, and if we care more about what they think than what we know and how we feel, we're abdicating our Free Will. As a result, in childhood many of us got our Instrument Panel completely out of whack and couldn't navigate anymore. "I love this, but mom says it's bad," or "This feels bad to me but my teacher says it's good." Up was down and down was up—which way do I go to feel better?

Some of us unplugged our Instrument Panel, numbed out, or ignored its signals, put a big fake smile on our face, and marched on, continually surprised at the things that happened to us that didn't make any sense because we didn't feel them coming. We had no clue how we got there since we couldn't feel the Instrument Panel readings.

When you go slower and stabilize at each new higher altitude, Law of Attraction supports you, you don't fall back, and you eventually stick at a new, higher set point. Because of the "sticky effect," the mind rejects affirmations that are too far from what you now believe; the leap from depression to joy is too big to sustain it. If you say, "I'm skinny and healthy," but your feelings say, "You're lying, you're fat," you're trying to make too big a jump. Go for a more modest jump you can "buy," such as: "I'm practicing raising my vibration every day." Cheery talk that you don't "buy" doesn't raise your altitude; it just fools you into thinking you're tipping the nose up when you're not, and the ground is still rising to meet you. Take it step by step.

While I didn't fully understand Law of Attraction back in those days, I now realize how it factored into the dilemma with the attorney. The sticky effect of my old vibration made it difficult to leap up to making that much money at once from one project. On the subject of money I had a mixed vibration: victim mixed with confidence. I had just finished some work where I'd felt disempowered. Now I remember feeling nervous when the attorney first gave me the work. My head was saying, "Oh, yeah, I'm confident. I have the job—this is good, ignore those fears." while my gut was vibrating, "Something's not right here," but I didn't know what it all meant. Today, I would never ignore a feeling and say, "Feel the fear and do it anyway." Yikes! I would either raise the vibration first before taking it on, or not do it. Your real power comes when you begin to feel what you're attracting *while you're attracting it,* and so have time to raise your altitude in time to change it.

Practice until you can hold a high vibration about something you want. Soften and allow the sticky contradictory feelings and thoughts to be until they rise. When you can enjoy that higher feeling for just a few minutes without contradicting it you are on the way to mastering attraction.

You're never standing still—you're either very subtly spiraling upward or downward at any given moment, since Law of Attraction is always compounding *whatever* you're vibrating. But Grace is always lifting you and offering its upward momentum if you'll allow it in.

Blind Spots

WHILE GRACE DOES supersede Law of Attraction and gives you unearned boosts in altitude, you can be sure Law of Attraction isn't ever cheating you. We're never victims. Life does make sense. Even if I don't know *how* I created something, as soon as I can muster it, I *claim* I created it, because saying I didn't create it makes me a victim.

I don't *blame* myself for creating unwanted things: that's *self-victimization*. I take responsibility, not blame, and that restores my power instantly. I can use that power to move forward and create something else.

When your vibration on a subject is high, but you still haven't received what you want, you're either taking score too soon, vibrating lack, or broadcasting energy you're not aware of. I call that a blind spot. You've been practicing some vibrational habits for so long you don't know you're doing it. You've stopped feeling it, stopped noticing that it feels bad—or you unplugged your Instrument Panel. You've become numb to certain things or have come to accept that they are "normal." Feeling bad is *not normal*.

We "bought" beliefs and vibrations in our early years and now they may be invisible to us. Whole cultures and families vibrate things unconsciously, like prosperity, violence, unworthiness, poverty. Or peace, love, confidence, and worthiness. If you don't choose awakening, the world pulls you in random directions. When we're living in limited, constricted beliefs, it's hard to see what's possible outside that. It only occurred to me after Divine Openings just how extremely warlike America is as a collective. Some countries don't fight; it's just not in their collective consciousness or cultural beliefs. Some countries have a victim vibration, and get abused by other countries, or their own leaders.

Divine Openings gradually opens your eyes to blind spots you couldn't see before. Get Divine Openings help if you suspect you have blind spots.

Unconscious broadcasts or blind spots attract, too.

YOUR SECOND Divine Opening: You don't have to relate to nor deify this Thai Buddha to get the benefit of this Divine Opening. I've never studied Buddhism or eastern religions. I've never been a "path follower." I am a universal human. This painting just flowed out of my paintbrush after looking at a statue of a Thai Buddha during a road trip. It was painted outdoors on a picnic table in a California RV park.

Each Divine Opening is unique and it won't be like your last. You don't have to feel anything during any Divine Opening for it to work powerfully at levels below your awareness. Don't work or try. Just allow Divine Grace.

Divine Opening

This work of art opens a vortex of Grace and activates your consciousness.
Sit quietly and contemplate the image for two minutes.
Then close your eyes and lie down and feel
for at least fifteen or more minutes.

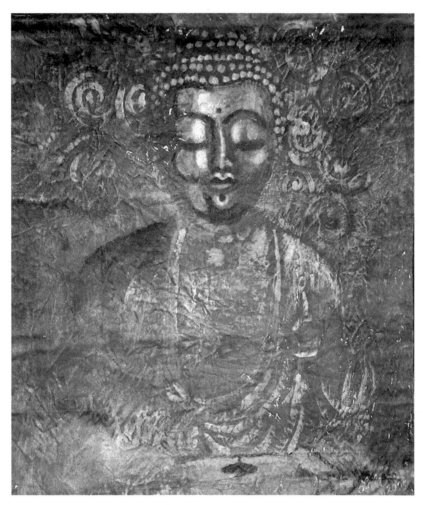

Figure 3—Thai Buddha, *a painting by Lola Jones.*

You Create What You Focus Upon

EVEN THOUGH DIVINE GRACE is lifting you up, you can use your Free Will to go with the flow of that Grace, or you can resist it. Your focus and attention is as powerful as any guided missile navigation system. When you consistently focus upon what you want, it's like pointing the nose of your missile toward it. You end up where you're pointed. Focus on where you want to go and you arrive there in good time. Each time you detour (complain to yourself or friends, tip the nose down, talk about it not being here yet, or indulge in negativity) simply remember your desired destination: look for what's good, imagine you're there, get in Large Self perspective, and refocus. Soon you're back on track.

I used to live six miles from the airport as the crow flies. I could see it from my hilltop. But I had to drive fifteen miles to get there—there was no road straight through to the airport. Life is like that sometimes. Just take the road you're guided to take and stay focused on the destination, not worrying about the twists and turns of the indirect route. Even if you get off course, your Large Self, your internal GPS, recalculates your route, so you can't really fail as long as you keep moving.

When you consistently focus upon what you don't want, it's like saying you want to go to California, but then pointing the nose of your plane toward your old house in New York. Pointing toward the old house, talking about how crowded and noisy the old neighborhood is, and complaining about how you keep ending up in New York keeps you in New York.

In life, focusing on what you don't want and expecting to get what you do want is insanity. Even if you have very real physical evidence of the unwanted reality that you always end up in New York, you can't afford to focus on it. Focus so intently on what you want that you drown out all contradictory vibrations. Then the essence of what you want *must* come. But don't get tense about *when* it's coming, or a specific form it must appear in—that increases resistance! Tension = resistance. Enjoy life, appreciate what's already here, and stay soft and open to all possibilities—that reduces resistance.

Most humans keep looking at the unwanted thing and give their power away to it, unwittingly feeding it their energy. The wife is not doing what the husband wants her to, so he thinks about his dissatisfaction all the time, and that story spins up more dissatisfaction. Her behavior magnifies from his attention to it, they fall out of love, and they divorce. Terrorism exists, so our leaders encourage us to fear it and focus on it, which increases our insecurity and fear. War is real, we don't like it, and we want it to go away. So we talk about how bad it is, we read about it, protest it, join groups who oppose it with us, and argue about which politician's fault it is. We become generators of fear and aggression. The good news is that each of us affects the collective powerfully by raising our own consciousness. A highly enlightened person offsets and balances the collective consciousness energy of millions of lower vibration people. High vibrational energy is exponentially more powerful than the same amount of lower vibrational energy.

The nature of Life is constant change and everything in our lives is constantly moving. It doesn't get stuck, we do, by recreating the same things over and over by vibrating the same way over and over. Reality never really stands still, so you can turn it on a dime if you stop vibrating the same old thing. Disease would heal itself and money situations would improve naturally if we congruently vibrated health and prosperity. When we obsessively look at disease and debt, we literally keep creating the same thing over and over again as our attention feeds our own power to it. When you're hooked by something really strongly, notice you're pouring your gas into its tank—draining your tank all the while.

After working with thousands of people, I noticed that most who were in therapy were constantly creating *more* issues and unpleasant feelings—*by talking about them.* After taking our Certified Guide training, therapists teach them to drop the story and feel the feeling. To soften into the feeling and allow it. The Grace this book offers makes it easier, and those therapists give this book to their clients.

You're always "manifesting." The key is to wake up to HOW you're doing it.

If someone says, "But I need my outer reality or this person to change before I can feel good." I say "Uh-oh, you're in trouble now! That's backwards. Find the feeling you want now." How empowered are you if your environment, other people, and outer circumstances can determine how you feel, and create your reality? When you choose your focus, no matter what is going on, no matter what anyone else is doing, no matter what your circumstances are—you are free and powerful. Claim your power to create whatever you want, from wherever you find yourself. I want my nose tipped upward independent of what anybody else is doing or saying. When I'm up here, I can help others get up here, too.

Just on principle, don't let anyone cause you to feel any way that *you don't choose.* That's the most important power you have—to choose your attitude and your altitude. Claim your power, and *decide* to keep your vibration up independent of everything else. Nothing is worth dropping your vibration.

The most famous, and most extreme story of the power to choose is told in Victor Frankel's book, *Man's Search for Meaning.* Frankel survived a Nazi concentration camp with his heart open. He determined that he would remain loving, care for others, remember his purpose, and keep his thoughts focused on living, even amid constant daily evidence of meaninglessness, cruelty, and death. His young wife and child perished, but his power to choose his reality remained steadfast, enabling him to live on to marry again. Together they taught others how to choose their own thoughts, feelings, and attitudes. He refused to hate his captors, so he never closed off *his flow of love* nor lost his alignment with God.

The key to creating what you want is to focus on what you want, then let go, and do your daily best not to contradict it. Then the Law of Attraction must bring it to you. If the unwanted thought or reality grabs your focus again, quickly pivot. A good mantra for this:

Nothing is worth lowering my vibration!

Don't fret about your lower thoughts and feelings—don't resist your resistance! Your positive thoughts are more powerful than the negative ones, and the dominant force of Grace in the universe is on your side. Don't worry about being perfect—you don't need perfection. You only manifest seriously unpleasant things when you give a lot of energy to low vibration thoughts for quite some time.

Habitually happy people have consciously or unconsciously trained their biochemistry to be happy. Train your mind by practicing good-feeling thoughts. Say to yourself, "I will feel good no matter what." Be so dedicated to feeling good, and so committed to being in alignment with your Large Self, that you always find some way to feel just a little bit better in spite of *any* outer condition. What other sane choice is there?

Most people think when they describe a situation they're reporting *facts*. But when you *describe* it, you start *vibrating* it, then you're actively *creating it*. Your story about it spins up a vibration, and vibration creates reality. Be conscious of your words, your stories, what you give your attention to, and what you create! When people tell their stories in sessions, I remind them, "It doesn't matter how much evidence you have that it's true. The only two things that matter are—does that story point the nose up or down, and is that the direction you want to go?"

Soothe yourself. When you observe something you don't want, soothingly say to yourself, "Everything always works out. This is temporary. It will change. All I want is coming to me. Might as well feel better now, in the process." Some people learn to self-soothe by hearing me demonstrate it. There's an audio set called Soothe Yourself, on the website under Talk Audios.

Stop letting what you observe "out there" dictate your feelings and your reality. If you let "the facts" dictate your vibration—you're a victim. Claim your power and be a creator rather than a reactor, observer, or reporter of "facts." Choose the way you want to feel—it creates the reality you live in.

Others may not understand your choices and may even accuse you of not caring for them if you won't commiserate with them in the lower altitudes, but you do the most good in your world when your altitude is high. You cannot help anyone at all when you go down there. Let them know you love them, listen to what they say and feel, but don't go down there with them. I don't preach or teach outside of class. I just listen compassionately, nod, and shower them with love. I don't go down there. People who want you to suffer with them may say, "You're being selfish!" With compassion and humor, you can say, "You want me to feel bad with you? Who's being selfish?"

Focus on what you want. Rave about what's right.

Everything simply will not fit into this book, and even if it would, it's best to stabilize at one level before going higher. *Watch Where You Point That Thing: Mastering Your Power of Intention*, the book that follows this one, is completely different Level 2 material that guides you much more deeply into how to master your power of intention—how to use your focus as a powerful laser beam that etches and carves your reality.

Worthiness

YOU EXIST. You were given life. Therefore you are worthy. Period. End of subject. You're part of the All That Is, so you're worthy. You have possibly been working too hard to attain something you already have, or to prove something that was never in question—your worth. Unworthiness is a mind-construct.

Unworthiness doesn't really exist. Even people you think of as bad or evil are worthy, as The Divine gave them life and Free Will to do anything they choose. Yes, Hitler went back to pure positive energy, or Heaven, just like Mother Teresa. The Indweller does not judge what you choose to do with your gift of Life, but generously gives Free Will to all, knowing there is no ultimate risk for an eternal being. Mistakes don't exist either, and are not tallied by The Divine nor held against you. Karma is a primitive religious concept, much like Hell and damnation. They both deny Grace, and you can let go of them now. Each life, each day, each moment, is a fresh new start.

Life is about inner freedom, happiness, and love—if you'll allow it. We are here to live, laugh, love, enjoy, create, expand and choose whatever we want. There is nothing to earn, get, overcome, or prove. Many people concluded that if they had been worthy, they would have gotten the love and care they wanted, the popularity, or the good stuff. It had nothing to do with worthiness. We have mistakenly transferred human qualities onto God. For example, when our parents or other humans judged us instead of loving us unconditionally, we concluded that God is the same way. Human love is fickle and conditional. Divine Love is unfailing and unconditional. Your Large Self, adores you no matter what.

Religions sometimes tell us we are unworthy, and if you believe it's true you will live the consequences of that belief. Our beliefs play out in our reality, making them seem all the more real because "proof" always shows up to match our beliefs.

You learned unworthiness from other people who were separated from their Large Selves. They "proved" that belief over and over, and you may have bought it. You took on vibrations from them in order to be like them, to fit in and be safe. This happened so long ago that you don't remember doing it. You get accustomed to it, and don't question it, and you can't feel how damaging it is. If it feels bad, it's not your Divine state—you're out of alignment with what God thinks about it. Unworthiness feels bad, and it should, because it indicates your separation from God *on that subject*. The Presence loves you, and when you disagree and say you are unworthy, you are out of alignment with The One who created you.

Feelings of unworthiness are one of the biggest blocks to receiving Divine Grace, so the sooner you can release those judgments against yourself, the more fully you can receive the good that is flowing to you and through you all the time. Unworthiness is a lie and a mistake. Let it go. Decide you are worthy right now! God already has. Why not agree and get back in alignment?

The many pleasurable processes and the Grace of Divine Openings will help you *know* your worthiness and let in the unlimited good that's meant for you. Just be willing.

Worthiness is a given. You may let in all the good now.

The four most common resistances that slow down one's liberation are:

1) Unworthiness—You don't let the good in if you don't believe you're worthy of it.

2) Addictions—They usurp your will, use your power, and skew your choices. Release them.

3) Love that's not flowing with all people in your life, current and past. We address this later.

4) An over-dominant analytical mind. Let me sing Grace into to your soul, because you'll never, ever get Divine Openings with your brain. It just isn't capable of containing or explaining it. It can only shrink it.

It's your life and you're important.
Prioritize your evolution and all the rest comes.

What Was My Secret?

People have asked me why I came home with more freedom and power than others who participated in that very same twenty-one day retreat. I invite you to slowly *feel into* each one of my answers. These answers also explain why I can now get people to that same place in only five days in my retreats:

1) I gave no power away to anyone and focused solely inward, on The Presence, in the silence.

2) I let go of everything I knew, and became empty to make room for a completely new, upgraded life. Vast new power is found when you let go of everything and start fresh. Life got really simple.

3) I didn't try to figure it out, but went into No-mind and No-thing, a very powerful state of pure being, beyond rational thinking, beyond physical reality, pre-manifest.

4) I stopped seeking, grasping for answers, working on myself, and modality mixing.

No More Working On Yourself!

BEFORE I GIVE you more methods, I want to make sure you've completely let go of working on yourself—so you don't stuff Divine Openings into that tired old "work on yourself" paradigm and diminish it. Those years or lifetimes of working on yourself, learning "lessons," clearing karma, or healing yourself are the polar opposite of Divine Openings. Not wrong, but opposite. Sometimes it takes a while for readers to let it in, and repetition is good learning theory.

It really is possible to enjoy the Divine Openings processes, soften into them, let The Presence (your Large Self) do the work, and *that's it*.

Soften around the issues and problems, *focus on them less,* and whatever you're struggling with lifts or shifts naturally as you go. Divine Openings is full of resistance-melting Pleasure Practices—not work. If you work on yourself, or give your power to someone else to work on you, it delays or reverses your progress.

Here's the "cowgirl guru" in me speaking: Get a life. If your social life revolves around spiritual seeking, sessions, seminars, talking about issues, giving and receiving emotional support, processing each other, discussing new modalities, going to metaphysical meetings and meditations: *get a real life!* Share about this book, and soon friends and family will want to play with you, not talk about their problems, issues, what's wrong, or what they lack. Do real hobbies, and have fun. Get a life outside of work, too. Lighten up and live and all that seeking will start to feel really boring.

We all got on a spiritual path to get happy and have a great life, right? For so many seeking took over and became an end in itself—but it never ends!

You can begin to really live now.

Aren't All Energies the Same?

Someone asked, isn't all Divine Energy the same? No—while it's all Divine energy, you can observe that there are different frequencies of energy all over creation. Some frequencies are far more powerful than others, and they all produce different results. X-rays are different from microwaves. Would you try to cook with X-rays, or diagnose an illness with a microwave?

Although it's all radio wave energy, radio stations broadcast on many different frequencies and the stations are all completely different. Would you listen to two radios at once, even if both stations were great? Mixing different energies, books, and modalities is similarly chaotic and it confuses your vibration. When people are confused or unhappy and seeking, they tend to attract *more confusion*: more modalities, more books, which blocks the clarity and enlightenment they seek.

Keep it Simple

WHEN WE SEEK AND GRASP outside ourselves, which I did for twenty-five years, awakening is *impossible*. Our own guidance can be heard only after we stop drowning it out with too many voices and inputs. Your Large Self can get in the driver's seat only if you open a space for it there.

I'll never ask you to have faith or trust. *You only need faith when you have no proof.* When you practice Divine Openings you get plenty of proof. Make your own choices, please, yet those who get the big results say they kept it *simple, easy, and undiluted.*. That has certainly been the key to freedom for me. Since my silence twelve years ago, when I dropped everything except Divine Openings, I haven't worked on issues at all, but my pace of evolution has exponentially increased.

Truth is simple.

While I'd never make any other path wrong, long time Divine Openings students say most (not all) therapy, seminars, energy work, and emotional/spiritual "healing" modalities diluted the effectiveness of Divine Openings for them. Divine Openings points you inside, and opens you to know your own truth.

Energy work may make people feel better temporarily, but if they go back to the same vibrational habits and beliefs, and create the same conditions over again, it doesn't last. Moreover, by believing there's something to clear or heal, they unconsciously create things to get cleared or healed, and it *never ends*. It's a hamster wheel they never get off of.

Divine Openings isn't *"energy work."* It's not any type of "work." There is no therapy, cleansing, or clearing—no piecemeal tackling of endless issues. You can be *done* with that, yet your entire being will evolve automatically at a Grace-accelerated rate, directed by the Organizing Intelligence of your Large Self. That continues eternally.

Get clear on your choice: awakening—or endless seeking, fixing, and working on yourself.

We prefer to use the word "healing" only if you're physically ill. If you're not ill you don't need "healing work"—you only need to wake up. Neither you nor the planet needs "healing." Sorry, but some New Age stuff just keeps you on the hamster wheel of "there's something wrong with you and the world and you've got to fix it." Graduate from being a fixer to a powerful creator. Once free, you never have to go back, unless you get really sloppy and go back to sleep—or back to seeking outside yourself (same thing.)

Continue your exercise, yoga, bodywork, and massage. Simple meditations for pleasure are great—drop the complicated ones. Truth is simple. Practice your religion if it still speaks to you. You may read and listen to inspirational things, but if it's contradictory—has you "work on yourself," get fixed by or give power to someone else, "heal your emotions, soul, or spirit" (which are not sick and never were!)—that's giving your power away.

Now you can allow life to be simple.

What Is Compassion?

IF SOMEONE YOU LOVE fell into a deep well filled with water, with no way to climb out, what would you do? Would you jump in out of sympathy? If you did, what good would you do? What you'd probably decide to do is get a rope and stay up there in safety while pulling them out. It's the same with any deep dark emotional, spiritual, mental or physical hole that your friend or family member, community member, or nation finds itself in. Descending to that low feeling place doesn't help anyone out of it. It lowers your ability to be of any service to anyone.

In this process, focus on yourself for now. You can help others when you are liberated.

We got stuck with the odd idea that compassion is the same as commiserating, or sharing the burden. This has become so pervasive that people expect you to grieve with them, suffer with them, lament, and feel down with them. If you stay up, you are of more service to everyone, especially yourself. When someone is suffering, you can hear them and let them know you hear them, but don't go down there to that low place with them. Stay "up" no matter what is going on around you.

Compassion for yourself is primary. Before you read on, make a decision to be soft and easy on yourself. Many spiritual people have compassion for everyone—except themselves. Make peace with wherever you are right this minute, knowing you did the best you could, and that now you are moving forward, not looking back. Softening about where you are frees you to enjoy life on your journey, right now, today, just as you are. You are where you are! God is not judging—why are you? Are you as compassionate to yourself as you are to others?

Whatever you experience in this process is perfect. Enjoy the bliss, allow the lower feelings, and keep going. Give yourself lots of encouragement and support in this and in every area of your life. As the very entertaining Cajun minister Jesse DuPlantis said, "If you're going through Hell, don't stop! Keep moving!" This quote is from me:

"Heaven is just ahead."

Evolution Was Leading You to NOW

ALL THE SPIRITUAL STUFF you learned in this lifetime before you came to Divine Openings was not necessary to help you "get" Divine Openings at all. Beginners often get Divine Openings *faster* because they come empty and uncluttered. Previous study can be a handicap if the mind is attached to old stuff you "invested in" that didn't end your seeking.

But in the larger sense of human evolution you've been leading up to this place and time for lifetimes and eons, despite the detours. Life Force spent billions of years evolving this environment for You. Then it evolved You. You continue to evolve You, and will for eternity if you are willing. Source loves to create and expand, and never stops, so allow that evolution and it will unfold without working at it. You will never be done, so you can stop being concerned with perfection, completion, being behind, or "getting to enlightenment." Enjoy this moment as if it is Christmas Eve and you are about to open another astounding pile of never-before-seen gifts.

This moment is all there really is. This book is about becoming happy in this moment, and when you are happy in this moment, you are in agreement with The Presence. The time for enlightenment is NOW. The time for mankind to wake up is NOW. The methods are right here for you, right NOW, in this book. You are NOW on your way to enlightenment. Really! Finally.

Savor the journey. It's been a long time coming. On my spiritual path, for decades it seemed it would never come, but it's here now. It requires little from you, because by Grace it is given to you. Universal Intelligence is intervening and giving it to you where you were not able to find it or figure it out from study, logic, analysis, and limited human intelligence.

It has always been so. Monks of old would fervently study, pray and give devotions and service for years with no sign of enlightenment, and then one day, if they were fortunate, Grace opened them up instantly out of the blue. Divine Openings opens you to let that in *NOW*.

This moment is a new beginning, and eternity is full of endless new beginnings.

Many Personalities

YOU ARE NOT one single personality--you are many. Just observe them as they come and go in response to circumstances. At times you might be the taskmaster, the loafer, the child, the perfectionist, the fearful one, the miser, the leader, the follower, the dreamer, the lover, the nurturer, or the judger. Resisting unwanted aspects of yourself only strengthens them. Witness them as they come and go, observe them as *energies,* and embrace them all. Awareness is all you need to over time become more your authentic core self. Don't get caught up in fixing or processing them. That's playing their game, you'll never win, and it will never end. Let them flow without resistance and they move on, as all energy wants to do.

There may be times that you loathe yourself as you feel aspects of you that are far separated from your Divinity. You may feel embarrassed, guilty, shamed, or disgusted by things you've said or done one day, and superior to others the next. Be with the feelings, and drop the story about what you did. Feel with no words. Really, that's all you need to do. The Presence adores you no matter what and is not judging you. Once the feelings move, your vibration rises.

I never talk about ego. The ego is an artificial construct that doesn't really exist, and struggling with any illusion is insane. You need a sense of separate self to ensure your survival in the physical plane. People with what are labeled "big egos" are responsible for some of the most beneficial discoveries and events in history. Don't make it wrong, and don't worry about it. What you resist persists. Just focus on being your Large Self, and you'll have no need to be concerned with ego. Your small self naturally refines as you unfold. It may go through stages, from "I'm worthless" to "I'm better than everyone" to a more mature appreciation of *your authentic magnificence.*

Who or What Is the Divine Presence?

THIS IS NOT a religious book. Anyone with an open mind, of any faith, or no faith at all, will benefit from reading it and from the awakening they receive from it. Although I use terms like The Divine, you can substitute Universal Intelligence, the Organizing Intelligence, The Indweller, Source Energy, The Creator, The Presence, The Light, Jesus, Buddha, Mohammed, Quan Yin, The Mother, Gaia, Nature, Life Force, It, The Absolute, The "I Don't Know What It Is," Fred, or any term you like.

It doesn't matter what you call it, it knows exactly who it is! And you will experience it for yourself in this process rather than taking my word or anyone else's second-hand word about it. That said, I will share my perceptions, which are of course filtered through my current state of consciousness and are the highest vibration I had access to when I wrote this. It keeps evolving, and the newest downloads I get can be experienced in the Online Course Portals and live retreats.

Will we ever know the full extent of The Divine Mystery while we are in these bodies, using this brain? Will we define it with words and scientifically nail it down? I doubt it. You'll have plenty of opportunity to know that mystery fully again after this life, when you return to the vast unlimited being you were before this life. But I want you to feel and know it NOW, in this body, *in this life.*

A physician who professed no belief in God took a live course series with me. Atheists don't usually come to me, and I was curious to find out what she would experience. Her eyes lit up and began to shine after her very first Divine Opening—the Presence in her was waking up very fast. It was funny; she had no context for her experience, and it confused her. Something was happening. There was something inside her that she had not believed was there—yet there it was! She had no label or explanation for it but it was real. She looked stunned. She darted in and out of class without saying anything, until later, when she'd email me of the changes in her life. She was uniquely blessed in having a direct, authentic experience of The Presence without the baggage of past cultural conditioning, religion, and dogma.

Her pervasive anxiety about life, relationship, career, and single motherhood disappeared after the first class. Gone. That too can be a bit disorienting for people. When a feeling they've felt their whole lives is gone, it may feel like a void, or even a loss, but it's soon filled with something better.

Whether you believe in it or not, it's already there inside you, and you will experience it.

"Experienced" and "advanced" people, the more you let go of all preconceived notions, the more purely you can experience The Presence directly rather than through tired old concepts and filters.

With Divine Openings, we experience a very personal God directly, and most of us lose interest in talking about it, preferring instead to just be in it. Definitions and labels only shrink it to fit inside the limited human brain. People often say to me after a Divine Opening, "It's difficult to explain." I can only smile and nod.

The Creator has levels of being, from the most infinite and large aspect that is indefinable and unknowable to us, down to the most personal aspect that has descended into materiality as us. That largest aspect is impersonal, and frankly, I don't think it is concerned with us; the universe on that scale goes on with or without us. Nobody misses the dinosaurs. It is the more personal, relatable aspect of God that we focus upon and cultivate here.

The Divine Presence, or our Large Self, is always in bliss, and has no judgments about any of our experiences. The Divine knows its (and our) eternal nature, so death, destruction, our wrongs, errors, and seeming tragedies are flickers on the eternal screen of life. The Presence within us hums along at its high, fine vibration no matter what is going on in our human lives. Whether we humans awaken or not, and no matter how our lives go, from its high vibration, the Essence Of Life enjoys and expands by living through us. God never dips down into the lower vibrations as we do, no matter what happens. The Presence always sees infinite possibilities, offers solutions, and holds the vibration of the solution for us as a steady homing signal. We came here knowing we would be able to experience lower vibrations and contrasts: joy and suffering, fulfillment and frustration, enthusiasm and despair, feelings we like and ones we don't. If it you can't yet consciously choose among the contrasts, keep practicing—you will get it.

There is much more to you than you see, yet it's not always so easy for you to know, since you use your physical senses to decide what's real, and your physical senses cannot always perceive the Non-Physical. But your Large Self—that vast, unlimited, Non-Physical aspect of you of which you are but a small physical aspect—is always there for you, and you can know and feel it intimately.

Many of you reading this book already accept that you have lived before this, that you lived before this physical experience, and you will live after. But the good news is that you don't have to die and go back to the Non-Physical to experience that broader Non-Physical aspect of you; you can experience it right now. Wondrous guidance is available to you through this Inner You that has the full view of reality at all times—the all-encompassing perspective of your Larger Self.

A student sitting in my seminar room, seeing my Divinely inspired painting of a Thai goddess (you'll see it later in this book) asked if I had past lives in the East. Sure, that goddess was me, but all that I became in past lives is here with me NOW, and becomes even more expanded each day without "doing anything." I don't go back in time to seek or discover anything. As I counseled her, the Goddess smiled from the wall, but that energy and wisdom are within me here and NOW. I don't plan sessions or even five-day retreats. It comes through in the moment as I relax, let go, and allow the flow.

Your Large Self calls to you to wake up and remember all that *you* are—to experience life as your Large Self does, wise, joyful, with acceptance and compassion, without judgment, without suffering, without struggle. Your Large Self emits a constant homing signal, calling you to come home, to live powerfully and magnificently as The Presence in physical form.

It's not "healing," it's "waking up."

I was deeply honored when I saw my place in creation—at the center of the universe. Of course, wondrously, everyone else is also at the center of this holographic universe. Co-creating with The Creator, we get to amend, adjust, and improve it to our liking.

The formless, Non-Physical Essence Of Life needs you and me to fully experience the wonder of physicality. When you walk this earth fully awake as your Large Self, knowing that you are a physical point of focus of The Divine, The Creator's desire to play full out in material form is fulfilled. You trek into new frontiers, and create things that have never before been. As eternal beings we are never finished, and The Creator is never finished expanding and experimenting. Let go into this vast, endless adventure with a deep relaxing breath!

The Divine can't do it without you!

People talk about finding their purpose, as if it's some serious, weighty thing. It is such a Puritan ethic to think God has some big heavy expectation of you, or that to be complete you have some mission to accomplish. Nothing could be a bigger distortion of the truth. Your purpose is to enjoy your life! Discover and let go to who you really are—your Large Self, a joyful being—and your talents will multiply and expand without trying. "Life purpose" is a silly New Age notion. Ask a giraffe what its purpose is. Its purpose is to live. I guarantee messages from your guides saying you must fulfill some heavy mission are filtered through some old, outdated concept of God. You are the hands, voice and body of The Divine, but lighten up about it. Love, live and enjoy. Serve if it really feels good to you. Playing actually adds just as much value to the planet as work does.

A few people will not be able to hear what I'm saying. They might even get angry at me. When feelings begin to move some will run like hell. A few years before I met her, a friend had quite a flashy cosmic oneness experience—one you'd probably think was the ultimate. But her awakening didn't last, because she wasn't willing to feel lower vibrations, nor accept that she creates her life. "I didn't create my ex-husband . . ." "My dad is just an idiot. . ." I could only smile when she said about this book, "That book makes me feel things I don't like." She quit reading it. (We remained friends.)

Every teacher, medium, channel, psychic, indeed every human being, hears, sees, and feels different things when they talk to God, depending on their level of consciousness. The thing that is "true" at one level of consciousness is "less true" at a higher level of consciousness. It is very challenging to experience God fresh and uninfluenced by cultural images and myths, but I encourage you to aim for it. Your understanding of God evolves endlessly with Divine Openings.

I share with you insights about Life from my own experience and inner knowing, and it continues to evolve, as yours will. Your understanding of Life is filtered through your current level of consciousness. What you "hear God saying" will always be colored by your vibration and your beliefs.

When someone says God said something angry, harsh or judgmental to them, that they got bad news from God, or that they experienced some negative manifestation of Spirit, that is the highest voice they can hear at that level of consciousness. You cannot watch channel 24 television while your dial is tuned to the channel 7 frequency. You are getting the highest level input you can from where you are at all times. Soften. Be willing to let go of what you "knew" last year. *That's already out of date.*

The authors of the ancient texts wrote at their current level of consciousness, and each translator after them colored their interpretation with their own consciousness, often with strong political or religious control agendas. It's easier to control people who don't know their true magnificence.

A teacher or medium with unresolved anger vibrations will hear an angry God and pass that message to her students. A teacher who has unresolved fear vibrations will channel messages of danger, violence, entities, evil spirits, and apocalypse, and urge you to take protective measures. A person with active sadness vibrations will give less positive messages about love and relationships. In my twenty-one days of silence and solitude, I deliberately let go of all my past conditioning, emotional baggage, preconceptions, and spiritual concepts so I could more purely experience The All That Is.

To even be able to hear what I'm saying, you have to have space in your mind for it. You must be in the vibrational neighborhood of this material. Some people slept with the book under their pillow for a long time until they were ready to open it. Often a person who didn't get it at first picks the book up again and says, "Why didn't I get this before?"

As I look back on my own evolution, I see how my view shifted with my consciousness. I wrote a book called *Dating To Change Your Life* long before I created Divine Openings. It was a breakthrough for me and it helped many people. So many of those ideas, rules, and beliefs no longer applied after Divine Openings. But for people at that level of evolution with relationships, the book is still a hugely valuable, life-changing experience! Life attracts the right people to each book.

One universal quality of a high-level teacher is simplicity. If the method or the message is very simple, direct, and effective, it is usually of a higher vibration. If it is complicated, technical, difficult, and you need the teacher's guidance at every turn, it is not liberating you. The Divine needs no complicated processes, theories, or methodologies; its workings are elegantly easy, efficient, and fast if you allow it to be.

Personally, I respect teachers whose message has a very high and positive vibration; I avoid doomsayers and purveyors of bad news. Although I most often go within for guidance, information, or inspiration, I take inspiration from any messengers The Divine sends, regardless of their station in life. A friend, passing stranger, or street person sometimes delivers a surprise gift from The Divine. These synchronicities are appreciated even more as we recognize that in the Oneness the "others" who are bringing the messages are aspects of ourselves. Increasingly, I experience myself as an aspect of The Presence.

Design Your Own Unique Relationship with The Presence

BECAUSE THE VAST All That Is, the ultimate form of God, is so large, unknowable, and impersonal that we cannot possibly relate to it, our best way of "knowing" God is to create a more personal, relatable form that we can talk to. Going inside for your answers becomes easier when you can relate intimately to The Indweller, and when you can translate its pure vibrations to words you can understand. Man has sought relatable concepts of God since the dawn of consciousness, from the first Stone Age drawings, the rain and fertility gods, the many specialized Hindu deities, the Greek mythologies, the White Buffalo Woman of the Native Americans, Jesus, and so on.

This more personal God does know us, and does care about us, and wants not only our survival, but also our joy and thriving. This more personal God created us, and each of us is a holographic locus of it. That is why each of us feels like the center of the universe—indeed we truly are. In reality there is only one "Being" in many unique and wondrous bodies and forms, each with the illusion of being separate.

The Indweller is willing to make itself known to us in a form we can embrace or relate to. To a Christian, it may make itself known as Jesus, the Holy Spirit, or The Lord. To a Hindu, it might come as a specialized aspect like Krishna, Lord Ganesha, Lakshmi or Shiva. To a Buddhist, Buddha, although

Buddhists don't believe in a god, but in existence itself. To a New Age person, it may be a white light; to a more scientific type, a formless Universal Intelligence or order. For a musician it might be felt in inspired music. You may know it as the life force, intuition, or consciousness. Others call it Mother Nature. God doesn't care what name we call. Only man makes those kinds of ridiculous dogmatic judgments.

In India, a most remarkable thing happened to my concept of God. I realized that God has no self-nature, but is what you believe God to be, and that the amount of Grace you are able to let in depends on the relationship you have. I had seen evidence of this before in my devout grandparents on my father's side, who indeed did always get what they asked their God to provide, even down to physical healings and miracles. However primitive their evangelical Hell and brimstone beliefs seemed to me, they had a personal relationship with their God *that worked*.

As a child and a teen, I couldn't separate the good from the bad of it, and I couldn't relate to this judgmental God that my Assembly of God preacher grandfather talked about at all. We rob ourselves of infinite possibilities by holding onto inherited limiting concepts of God.

It was thrilling and inspiring to learn two new names for God when I was in India. While I never cared about Hindu traditions, these names forever changed my relating with The Divine, and helped me design a concept of God that I could actually walk and talk with like an intimate friend:

Yathokthakari: One who does as is bidden.

Bhakti Paradina: One who is at the beck and call of the devotee.

What a stunning concept—that God behaves according to our expectations and is actually willing to do what *we* want rather than dictating its will to us! It shouldn't be so surprising—reality bends itself to our beliefs.

While I thought I had already ditched those negative concepts of God in my thirties and embraced a more loving and inclusive God, I realized that the vast formless God I'd been trying to relate to was just too nebulous and impersonal, too conceptual for me to really connect with in any personal way.

No wonder the relationship had been cool and distant. Life is hot and close-up, and your God better be intense and real if it's going to compete with your daily in-your-face-physical reality. My God had been less real than the very distracting outer reality. I needed a God that was more up-close and personal. One of our challenges in the physical plane is to not let the material world dominate, or even become our God. Whatever has most of your attention, and whatever you give your power to—that's your God. When life circumstances are in your face, they can grab your focus and drown out your all-important internal God focus.

When we were children, naturally our image of our parents got transferred onto our image of God; not surprising—our parents *were* God to us—the conduit through whom all things seemed to flow for so many of our impressionable years. My father was an uncommunicative, strong silent type, so of course, my concept of God was like that. If your parents were non-judgmental and kind, encouraging and supportive, loving and wise, your concept of God is more likely to be like that. But if your parents were the average parents, you may need to toss out those less than positive unconscious perceptions of God and replace them with qualities you *want* in your God. Why? Because God behaves the way you expect, and life will bring you the consequences and the proof of your belief.

Since all this gets conditioned in us before we learn to use words, it can be invisible, hard to identify, so deeply ingrained that we don't even notice it. How could fish notice they are in water? No other reality is imaginable! You don't feel your clothes on your skin—you don't notice it because you've felt it all your life. We literally can't feel those early assumptions because we've never felt anything else and so have no contrast to compare them to. Most people never got the opportunity to clear that up—until now. It's not work, though. All you have to do is ask for Divine help, design your new concept of God, and God will do the rest. The Divine will even come to you if you are afraid of it, angry at it, or have doubts. Just ask.

I created a persona of God that I could really talk to and relate to; in effect, I designed my own ideal relationship with God, giving Him/Her all the qualities my heart desired, all the qualities my earthly parents didn't have, and all the support I had wanted from Life but hadn't received.

This was fun! I asked that "my" God relate to me with humor, playfulness, friendliness, and caring, in addition to all the expected qualities like unconditional love, all-knowingness, and power (but without being a bossy authority.) Later on I amended that to a God who cared about my every need, my every concern, who wanted to play with me and participate in every aspect of my life, who gives me messages I can understand, who loves to co-create with me, and who considers me a partner. God finally evolved into an inner friend who really listened and communicated back to me in feelings, Direct Knowing, occasional signs, events, or in my own inner voice. This was quite different from the old one-way pleas to the angry, petty, judgmental God my grandfather had preached about. Grandpa meant well, but had told me that God condemned girls wearing pants, and while I had not exactly bought it, it had distanced me from "that judgmental God" that felt so bad. The word "God" back then filled me with confusion and guilt. Many of you still feel that. Notice if you wince when you hear it. This new God needed me, valued me, and delighted in all my adventures, and even my mundane daily tasks. This continued to evolve for me until now I cannot even conceive of myself as separate from God, so it's hard to even call it a "relationship." Start where you are, talk to God constantly, and update it every year.

Many people still have resistance to authority figures, and if you do, guess what? God seems like the ultimate authority figure, which puts big distance between you and God without your knowing it's happening. Take God out of the authority figure role and put God into the nurturing role if you want a more open, loving relationship that supports you.

With help from Divine Openings, God becomes a tangible reality, an experience instead of a concept, and it begins with this redesigning process. A humorous miracle during my silence brought it all home to me. I had a tiny flashlight I hung around my neck after "lights out" in the dark dorm room. Its little metal handle broke one day, and one piece of the metal was lost.

I sat the flashlight on the dorm room nightstand overnight. The next morning the metal handle on the flashlight was fixed. It was whole; the missing piece had reappeared. There was no crack where the break in the handle had been. I laughed. My playful God had sent me a playful sign, and I understood. It said to me, "Everything is so assured for you now—there's nothing left for me to do for you but fix your flashlight." It also said, "Even this small detail of your life is so important to me that I will perform a miracle for you just to fix your flashlight." That tiny flashlight sits on my coffee table to this day, as a reminder. It brings tears of joy to remember.

If a voice inside feels good, I know it's my Large Self. If it feels bad, it's my small self. Minute by minute, day by day, my relationship with The Divine went vastly deeper than it had ever gone before.

The Presence will be whatever you want.

Soften around and eventually let go of any concept that you have to earn things, because if you hold that concept, you *will* have to earn everything. Decide that God wants to grace you with everything you want, with ease. Remember, worthiness is a given. Unworthiness is a human mind-construct. You are worthy just as the birds and flowers are worthy of their sustenance.

Soften and let go of and replace any concept that you have been judged as unworthy, because if you believe that, it shrinks your pipes, and Grace can't get in as easily. Decide to agree with God that your worth is already a given. The very fact that you were given the gift of life proves your worthiness. Simply reading this book and receiving the Divine Openings in it will help you open up to know your worthiness and let in the Grace that is offered to you in every moment.

Soften and let go of the belief that life is about lessons, because if you believe that, you will have lots of lessons, whereas if you believed life was about joy you'd have lots more joy. Life will evolve you, you'll learn and grow naturally, but this doesn't have to be some serious, dreary school! Decide that God wants you having fun as you evolve. You are actually closest to God when you're happy, and you'll soon know why.

Soften and let go of and replace any concept that your worldly needs and desires are not important to God. If you think your daily needs are trivial to God, you can't let as much Grace in. The Presence, of which you are an integral part, allows you to have what you want in the material world, so the more you can get out of the way and let that in, the easier it can be delivered. People who have their material and relationship needs met are freer to fulfill their spiritual lives. One who is constantly struggling to make ends meet makes neither a good model for others, nor has much time or money to have a spiritual life or to serve and uplift others.

Create a new relationship with a God who's up close and personal.

APPLY IT IN YOUR LIFE NOW:

1. **Write your updated concept of God in your journal,** or make a vision board of it. People who actually do these activities get the big results. Spend quality time talking to this new God, as you would build any new relationship. Continually update your concept of God as your consciousness expands. It will change.

2. **Read this article** and bust some old spiritual myths: DivineOpenings.com/spiritual-myths Click the Deutsch link for the German version.

Your Desires Granted

TALK TO THE INDWELLER within you constantly. Any kind of communication will work. It doesn't quibble about how you address it, or whether you call it prayer or meditation or conversation, whether you word it properly, or write down your desires or not. It's just happy to hear from you at all. Don't get hung up on words, processes, or rituals. Chat to God like an intimate, close friend. Be yourself. You can even argue with God or get angry at God. Who could handle it better or less judgmentally?

God is just happy to hear from you at all.

The Indweller knows your unspoken needs. When you feel bad, The Indweller hears that you want to feel good, and creates what you want. When you don't have what you want, The Indweller feels your wanting. I've had students spontaneously heal from long-standing injuries during Divine Openings when they had not even told me the problem existed, and they had not asked for healing. Divine Openings literally opens you up, so the Grace that's always flowing to you can get in. Many complicated healing and clearing technologies have been devised—not understanding how simple it is to ask and receive. Once Divine Openings has opened that door for you, you just feel what you need and want, soften around the feeling, and let go, knowing it's coming.

The basic formula is: ASK, ANSWER, ALLOW. You ask, The Indweller answers, you allow. Learning to soften your resistance, which gets you out of the way, is your main job, but it takes practice. The Indweller always hears you ask, even if you don't say it in words, even if it's just a discomfort you feel or a desire deep inside, so the asking is automatic on your part. The Indweller always answers yes, and grants the essence of your request, and just waits for the crack of an opening to fulfill it in the material world. Grace does 90%. Your only job, your 10%, is to soften around the desire, stay out of the way, and let it in.

Grace does 90%. Your 10% is to let it in.

Divine Openings helps you with the part humans have the most difficulty with: *allowing*, softening, *getting out of the way*, and *letting it in*. When our pipes are shrunken or rigid, Grace and good can't get in as easily. We ask and then don't let it in; we tense up, doubt, feel unworthy, focus on the lack of it, and so block its coming. Tension = resistance. Try this: tense up and clench your muscles, your jaw, your shoulders, ball up your fists. Imagine someone trying to give you something to make you feel better when you're like that. That's what resistance is. Now relax and hold out your open hands. Now you can receive with the aid of Grace. We can't fix it ourselves, but Grace can, without effort.

Just say yes. Say it out loud right now. *YES! YES! YES! Keep saying yes.*

I used to puzzle over why the Bible said that Jesus was the only way we could be "saved," since that seemed to exclude much of humanity who never heard about Jesus. I just could not see a loving Creator leaving anyone out. Now I feel it meant that man has trouble doing it for himself because he's so stuck in the small separate self, that the Grace of the Presence is the only thing powerful enough to do the job—

that the only way out of suffering for humanity is awakening with the help of that Grace. Mere action on the mundane level won't do it. You are "saved" (helped) by Grace, by any name. You will soon experience what that means, regardless of your religion or path. Divine Openings Certified Guides are trained to be "the hands and voices" that help bring that Grace down to Earth.

Many of us now have the sort of relationship with The Presence that allows us to simply think of something, without formal prayer or process, and that or something better comes. You can have that type of relationship too. This book shows how, step by step. Let go of any concepts of a God who doesn't support you; those beliefs block your receiving. When your God is loving, kind, and supportive, what you ask for is given, because it fits your concept of God. Your 10% is to let it in.

When your God is friendly and intimately involved in your daily life, the essence of everything you ask for, no matter how mundane, is delivered. People who have this type of relationship with God don't have to pray, or write it down, or set goals; they simply ask, and Life Force fulfills the request, just as any doting earthly father, mother, uncle, or benefactor would. You can have such a relationship when you begin to regularly talk to God like your friend and confidant, and stop thinking of God as some authority figure, separate from you. Now I'm at a place where I rarely ask for anything; I let go and let God guide me in the best directions. But yesterday I did ask for rain, and then let go. With no rain in the forecast, it came by this morning, and the week's forecast is full of rain. I never try to force or control—I ask lightly without attachment to the outcome, and let it go. If prayer feels intimate to you, pray, and know the answer is being given even if you know not yet what it is. The answer may not be a voice or a vision; it is more often a feeling, an inner knowing, a simple thought—or later, an event or person just shows up. Listen, watch, feel and appreciate it now—in advance—that speeds the arrival of it.

Take it Inside to the Presence

THE MAIN PURPOSE of my long period of silence in India was to spend all my time communing with The Indweller; to take it all inside to The Divine Presence—the feelings, the thoughts, the questions—to talk with The Presence and open that channel. I got answers (most were non-verbal), was nurtured, and developed that intimate relationship at a deeper, more tangible level than ever before. By avoiding even eye contact with people, I kept my focus inward.

It is delicious to be silent—the ultimate vacation! The growing relationship with my beloved Divine Presence within became too precious to even consider breaking the silence. It was like the intense first few weeks of a romantic relationship where your attention and focus is given only to the beloved, except this time it was the ultimate Beloved within.

The deeper into that silent embrace I dived, the sweeter it felt, and the stronger I became. It was ultimate fulfillment. My mind calmed down and stopped chattering and draining so much of my energy, and talking to others lost its addictive allure.

I noticed that those of us who took all our feelings, challenges and questions inside to The Divine had profound experiences, while those who turned outside to other people never developed that depth of communion with The Indweller nor tapped their internal power. Some of the participants could not bear the silence, and by taking their feelings and thoughts to other people or the monks they avoided deep feeling, didn't go direct to The Presence, and didn't claim their power.

Notice how trivial and ineffectual most talk is, how it leaks your energy, and takes you out of the moment. Notice how we use talking to run from feelings, even when we're talking about feelings! Talking about feelings was replaced with softly, silently feeling them all the way through. I lost my taste for counseling as I experienced an increasingly strong desire to take everything to The Presence Within. I marveled at the lightning speed with which my requests were being fulfilled. Once that inner relationship with The Indweller was established, the rest came easy. Things I had struggled with for years evaporated like mist. Divine Openings students eventually experience the same thing.

The Questions Cease

DURING THE TWENTY-ONE DAYS of silence, we were offered a half-hour each week to talk with the monks. Some participants asked many questions and hung on the answers, kids in a candy store stuffing themselves with goodies. Being so clear that I went there to find answers within, I was guided to begin to take my questions directly to The Presence instead. Answers to questions I had pondered for decades suddenly began to appear. For example, "Why had I become fearful years before when I saw a brilliant white beam of light in meditation, and again while out camping?" The answer came from within: the small self fears and resists everything unknown or unfamiliar. Images came to me of the Bible stories I'd read as a child where people fell down in fear and covered their eyes when confronted with an angel. Our small self is even afraid of our own brilliant light!

On about the ninth day, even my incessant internal questions to The Divine about life, love, money, the future, and the meaning of it all suddenly ceased—for the first time in my life. There was an eerie silence in my head. Rather than getting "answered," most of the questions simply lost their meaning or evaporated as my mind became empty, peaceful, still as a reflecting pool. I reported to the guides I had no more questions and respectfully didn't need to meet with them. I realized that most of our questions are just the mind doing its thing. The mind questions and doubts—that's just what it does. When the mind stops its chatter, and we are still, we can simply *be and know.*

All was quiet inside, and I would sit and marvel at the unaccustomed space inside my head. Any newly arising question was either answered immediately and definitively by The Presence Within, or were quickly recognized as unimportant mental jabber.

It became humorously clear that Life doesn't have a why. *Life is.* Life is for living, or as my friend Penny used to say, "Life just lifes." Asking questions, analyzing, trying to figure it out, naming and categorizing everything are mind-distractions from actual living. People who are truly living don't ponder the meaning of life—they live with gusto! They experience each moment. Ask a bird *why it lives.*

I would never have such big questions again. My questions are now practical. "What would make the most difference today?" "What would feel good?" "What will I create next?" "What's an easier way to get this done?" Now the answers just come, or I drop the question and let go till it does.

I became so empty that hours and days would pass with scarcely a thought rippling the surface of my mind. It was bliss. When I returned home to regular life, if my mind occasionally got cluttered, it cleared out again as I "laid it down at the feet of The Presence," and found stillness again. Soon a rhythm was established, thoughts came and went, leaving a clean slate for the next moment. This is truly the power of now!

When we have direct experiences of God, we don't ask questions about God; we are too busy experiencing it. Divine Openings gives you direct experience. Just live it and it all unfolds.

Cultivate your own direct knowing, and aim to go inside for most of your answers.

There had long been a desire to stop looking to any outer source for answers, comfort, information and direction. It was a dream come true. Once I was out of the way, The Grace that had always been raining down on me could finally get in. Everything I asked for came, some things in an instant, others in good time. Some things came in a different form than I expected. I became so confident that all things were coming that my old habit of doubting just *disappeared*. It never even occurred to me to work on myself ever again once I realized I was on an evolutionary fast track that required me to do nothing but pay attention and stay awake.

This habit of going within for most of my spiritual and emotional needs has persisted long since the twenty-one days of silence. The Divine is right here and will answer any need quickly, accurately and fully, from its unlimited resources and all-encompassing knowledge. All I have to do is soften and get out of the way. I might still ask for practical advice or help on matters of worldly expertise. The Divine sometimes sends an answer through another person. I still call tech support, although even for that, I might first close my eyes, still my mind, and receive inspiration; or get my vibration in receiving mode so I can let the help or answer in. Often the problem resolves itself!

How often do we give our undivided attention to The Presence for even one single day? That's why, even after leading over forty 5-Day Silent Retreats, I still cherish that time to focus within. Magic happens for me as well as the students, because there is always more, the deeper we go.

There is something you can always rely on, and it is right there inside of you.

There are still moments of confusion, and that means the old order in me is breaking down *yet again*, and I need to allow it time and space to rearrange itself. There is nothing to fix. A new consciousness opens up in good time, bringing with it new possibilities. Now, if confusion is caused by modality mixing, that will only clear up once you stop and refocus within.

Problems exist only in the consciousness that created them. In the brighter light of a new consciousness, the old questions often don't even make sense—they're non-issues. For example, when governments try to agree on what to do about nuclear weapons within the defensive and survival-based consciousness that created those weapons, all you get is treaties and regulations that partially work or don't work, and no one feels safe to follow them. In an expanded consciousness, people wouldn't even think of using those weapons. Questions of who should have what kind of weapons and how to regulate them seem pretty pointless from that new consciousness. We look back and wonder why it wasn't obvious before!

In most countries, a heightened consciousness about women has resulted in better treatment, equality and voting rights. The previous consciousness didn't support those possibilities. Suddenly, it seems very natural. Leaps in consciousness are birthed in a few people at first, in a few countries, then it spreads to others, then eventually, the entire material world changes to match. You are a front-runner for changes in consciousness. If it feels like it's taking too long, remember that evolution will go on forever. In the universal sense, there is no rush and no finish. Enjoy the ride.

When I returned home, help was always there for me, even if it was just a soothing feeling. The result was profound in my new work. Guidance poured in. Sometimes it was clear information, sometimes it was a feeling of, "soften around this, be happy, it will unfold." Sometimes it was a nudge to take action right now and the information poured into this dimension as I worked, typed, or spoke.

People asked me, "How do you know which thoughts are from The Divine and which ones are just noise?" I had not been able to answer that until I knew it from direct experience. Every one of us is constantly receiving communication, inspirations, nudges, whispers and suggestions from the Divine, but when our minds are loud and cluttered and our eyes are focused on problems and distractions, those inspired thoughts land in a din of thought-chatter, and sorting through that to find which thoughts are the inspired ones is difficult. The Divine usually whispers soothingly instead of shouting. Guidance isn't often delivered by a burning bush or a booming voice. But it became easy to recognize the subtle, quiet, Divinely inspired thoughts from inside my newly quiet, clear mind. Guidance always feels good, and it's always good news.

In the stillness you can hear the voice of God.
It usually sounds just like your voice, only smarter.

A Relationship with The Divine in Good Times

IN A CARTOON by Tex Reid, a cowboy walks into church and tips his hat to the preacher, who says, "What is it this time, Clem? Drought? Drop in cattle prices? Land taxes got raised?" After seeing how nurturing, how fun, how practical my new relationship with God was, I decided never again to relegate my communication with it to those times when I needed help. I knew God wouldn't judge me if I did that, but I would miss out. Now there is an ongoing, minute-by-minute dialogue, even when I'm communing with people, animals, and nature, working with my computer, or driving my car. God is everywhere and everything. Life is that communion. Meditation is great for the pure joy of it, or to simply rest in the deep silence of the Void. Meditation is more refreshing than sleep. Do it to reset, refresh or get empty, to merge with The Presence, but not to fix things or get somewhere.

People talk about meditating to save the planet. Get happy, radiate happiness, and that contributes high vibrations to the planet more than you know. Meditating from "there's something wrong with the planet," just creates more of that, and more discord in you. It can actually make it worse.

Although I'm usually naturally in the flow, some days I pre-pave my day, then let go so The Presence can line it all up for me, and so I can recognize the nudges and unexpected opportunities as they come.

Once I've asked for something I rarely ask again, because if it's not here, the only thing in the way is me—so I ask only for softening of resistance, and acceptance of the negative feelings about it. This creative, proactive focus has replaced the old fixing mindset, so problem solving and "healing" is no longer my life's focus. Sometimes I wake so clear about what to do that I just leap up and launch into it.

We are moving toward a new world that is based on *creation rather than fixing or problem solving*. Feel the difference. This is key.

Fixing, preventing, and surviving are of the old paradigm. We cannot see a higher solution while we're still in the same lower consciousness that created the problem. Our dialogues with God soon transcend asking for help (as child asks parent) and become more of a co-creative process (as with an equal.) The small self will tell you that you still need to keep seeking, working on yourself, and solving problems.

The mind is a wrong-seeking missile! It knows that once you are a free, empowered, creative being, the small self will no longer be in control.

Freedom from seeking and fixing is a strange and impossible concept for many, and it may seem incomprehensible at first. After a lifetime of struggle, overcoming, fixing, and earning, it may seem odd to simply hop on a new wave and be carried to wherever and whatever you want. What will life be about when you're not seeking enlightenment, striving to fulfill desires, trying to fix problems, or get somewhere—when all your basic needs are met? It's exciting to wonder, and out of that wondering will come your next steps.

If you could create anything you wanted, not out of need, but just for the joy of it (and you can and you will), what would it be?

Commune with The Presence in good times too! There are going to be a lot of them!

Second Chance for a Happy Childhood

ON ABOUT THE FIFTEENTH DAY of the twenty-one days I literally became a little girl again. I put my hair in pigtails, walked like a little girl, looked like a little girl, and felt as innocent as any fresh-faced child. When a woman walking by broke the eye contact taboo to laugh at my pigtails, I stuck my tongue out at her, and she giggled! I laughed at myself, realizing it was the authentic response of a five year old. I laughed again when Marian, who was seventy-four years old, stuck her tongue out at me a week later! We were had returned to innocence.

Splashing through puddles on the large lawn in front of the women's dormitory, laughing at frogs poking their heads out from the crevices, singing songs to myself, talking softly out loud to The Presence, it was a softer, gentler childhood than the first one. There was unconditional love and support, and this time the voice from within was soothing and wise. Unlike my first childhood, there were no voices inside or outside me to drown them out. Love had a chance.

There's an innocent child within you still.

Fear of the Unknown

YOU MAY HAVE a number of steps to take before you are ready to let go of some of your old vibrational habits, past hurts, working on yourself, and other baggage. Be soft and easy with yourself and appreciate, allow, and value your feelings. The less you push and try to fix things, the easier and faster it goes.

At one point it seemed the thing holding me back the most was my small self's fear of letting go of that last chunk of control. We know that our letting go to the larger flow of Life, or God—whatever you prefer to call it—is a key to freedom. The Ineffable Presence Within beckons us to turn our plane and go with the tailwind, but won't force us to, or take our Free Will away. The small self values its struggle and does not want to give it up because that's the end of its game. And it fears the unknown, even if it promises to be better.

We eventually let go and put the small self in the back seat while The Divine take the wheel. The small self may or may not throw little fits at times, just when you thought you had let go. But don't add more resistance to resistance! Be soft and easy on yourself.

Don't resist your resistance.

If you're struggling with fear of change, or of the unknown, simply soften around that feeling. Accept it best you can and allow it some space to be. Soothe yourself in kind tones. Take your attention off the story about why you have that feeling, and focus only on where the feeling is in your body, and what the sensations are. Breathe softly through it until you rise to acceptance.

The day after the twenty-one days of silence was over, we were all at the beach, resting, and I knew that the enlightenment process had begun but was far from over. I shared with Marian that I was still somewhat afraid of losing my small-self identity. She gave a snort, smirked, and said, "After seventy four years of it, I'm sick of it. I'll be happy to see it go!"

It was a pivotal moment for me; I could feel how in all her seventy four years, her small self being in control had never gotten her what she wanted. She was ready to let go to the flow of life. I didn't know which I was more afraid of, having my small self take a back seat, or having it keep driving!

My small self actually got very happy once I let go. It wasn't so scary after all.

Divine Opening

SIT QUIETLY and contemplate the image for two minutes.
Don't work or try. Just allow Grace. Then close your eyes and lie down
for at least fifteen to twenty minutes—longer if you can.

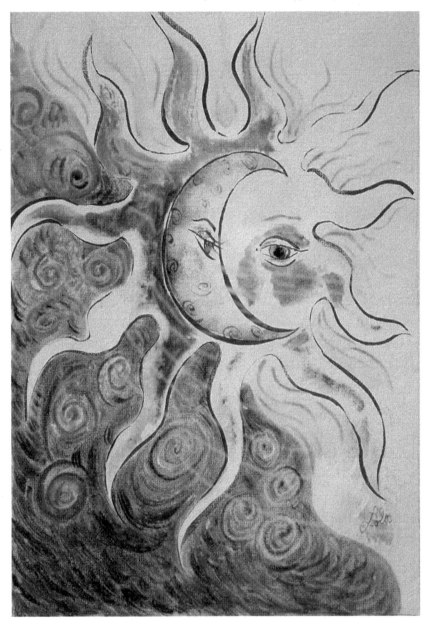

Figure 4—Solstice, *an ink drawing by Lola Jones.*

When Will I Be Done on this Planet?

WHEN I WAS a child I thought for sure I had landed on the wrong planet. I know many people who have felt out of place, and many who still do. "Who *are* these people who claim to be my family?" It is true that the earth plane can feel dense and heavy compared to the Non-Physical realm where the greater part of us lives, but once we know how this physical space/time reality works, its joys are great—so great that the Larger Non-Physical aspect of us clamors to come here repeatedly.

People only ask the question, "When do I graduate from Earth life and never have to come back?" when they feel separated from their Non-Physical Larger Self. When there is suffering, of course people wish for rest and deliverance. Once there is no suffering, there is no desire to leave here. Here is as good as anywhere. You got on the ride—now you get to enjoy it.

There is nothing to graduate from. There was never a test to pass. You don't earn your way out of here. That's that belief in "life as school" I was so happy to drop. When we know who we are and we are one with Divine Presence, we thoroughly enjoy this life, and are eager to return. You can skip school and go straight to the playground you so eagerly anticipated when coming here. You came here positive and full of plans, open and one with everything—now you can get back to that!

People who talk about wanting to ascend out of the body or who wish to leave this physical dimension have obviously not experienced the bliss of a fully awake body and a fully flowered heart! There is usually a lot of pain in their body and heart, so of course they want to leave it.

Along with many other spiritual myths we were told this body is somehow less spiritual than being Non-Physical. This time/space reality is on the leading edge of creation, it's "where it is at," and we are deeply blessed to be here at this time. There may be a time to move on to other dimensions of life, but when you do, it will be with the joyful farewell of a powerful and fulfilled being, not the retreat of a victim who has suffered enough. Enjoy this article: www.DivineOpenings.com/spiritual-myths (Also in German, just click the Deutsch button.)

It is inconceivable to ever imagine "finishing" anything in an eternal universe. When you live in bliss and peace and love you won't be worrying about fixing something in yourself or others. And you won't want to be rescued from this life—you will be truly living and enjoying it.

Life continues to flow in a never-ending stream of creation. You will increasingly create joyful and wonderful things, and then let them go. You will no longer resist anything or try to hold onto anything— you won't push it away and neither will you cling to it. One of the hallmarks of enlightenment is not just acceptance of or enduring what is, but authentically experiencing the beauty and perfection of what is. Of course, you cannot create this liberation with your mind, or pretend you feel it when you don't. Just soften, relax, enjoy the ride, and allow it to unfold. It will.

This time/space reality is the hottest game going, although it gets weary being here if we constantly try to fly into headwinds. Let go, let it take you, and it becomes a tailwind. After death we release all resistance. Then we line up bright and fresh to come back and give it another go, optimistic that next time we'll be able to remember, follow our inner knowing, and go with the flow instead of against it. From our Non-Physical perspective before we came into physical manifestation, we were eager to experience the wonders of physicality, knowing fully the challenges and possibilities of the game.

You can begin to enjoy this life now!

Part of the game here is to forget who we are, and discover it again—to go to sleep and then wake up. Babies love the peek-a-boo game where they cover their eyes, then peek through their hands. We are created in the image and likeness of our Creator, who also loves hide and seek games, adventures, and challenges. Most of all, The Creator loves to create.

True, once we get here and encounter the density of this plane, it can be hard to maintain the high vibration we started with. We encounter discord, confused energy, other people who are not aligned with Pure Source, and it's easy to get distracted. Trying to be like them so we'll be safe, we lose our fresh innocence, get bogged down and burdened by the thoughts and conditioning of society and other humans. It can seem like a bad idea to have come here.

As babies emerge from floating in the womb and feel the density of the material plane, their vibration drops a bit, and they cry. They're still quite open and One with Life Source. And then well-meaning people begin to teach them how to "protect themselves," what horrors to avoid, "how life works" and how tough it is. They lose their positive expectation bit by bit and begin to focus on things they do not want, and the downward spiral away from their Pure Essence begins. They lose their focus on their own inner knowing, start listening to other "more experienced" beings and stop trusting their own guidance. We start out knowing what feels good, then forfeit our own inner compass because it feels like we have to agree with others to be loved.

As a result, many people, especially spiritual people, begin to feel that they are "in the wrong place" or "on the wrong planet" or that this place is "bad" and needs fixing. When we return to the place of innocence and trust and connection, we are happy on this planet, with all its contrasting experiences, knowing we can choose, and that our safety is ultimately guaranteed. The "worst" that can happen to us is that we leave the body and return fully to our Non-Physical, unlimited, Large Self.

From that broader perspective, we relish Earth life, and are secure in the knowledge that even if we splat, we'll be back again for another ride, to take the evolutionary experiment on to yet another level. We know we can do even more next time because all of our desires that don't get fulfilled in this life carry over into the next. That's how evolution works. That's how the exponential growth of recent years happened. That's how kids recently born can use a computer by age three. Desires carry over from generation to generation to be fulfilled by a later generation, or use in a new body. The desires of past generations had built up to the point where a critical mass occurred. Even if they died before they ever got their desires, we're now reaping the benefits of that. The animal kingdom does this too.

After reawakening, you will not wish to be elsewhere. You'll be too busy living. The fully awake Divine Presence in you appreciates the opportunity to experience physical creation in the full sensory richness that only physical incarnation can provide!

You're in the right place! You can enjoy previous generations gifts to you now.

The End of Drama

VEILS LIFT AND things are seen that were invisible before, and there's no going back unless you get sloppy and forget. One unforgettable day long before Divine Openings came along, I remember having a flat empty feeling once there was no more drama in my life. I had ended an unhappy and dramatic relationship and begun a course of sane and proper dating with sane and suitable men. Looking back it was easy to see the old drama for what it was, and it was not pretty. The desperate "love," the fighting, conflict, complaining and commiserating, the longing and suffering and the extreme charge on those radical emotions now felt violent and unsavory to me. The small self douses life with a steady stream of inflammable fuel that perpetuates more drama. The endless conversations with friends to "solve problems" were just gasoline on the fire.

The evaporation of drama addiction left a void where before there had been zing and pop and zap. I didn't want it back, but I felt somehow lacking in what I had thought was passion. A teacher at the time told me that I could deliberately create a whole new kind of passion and excitement, comparable to developing a new taste for gourmet vegetable dishes when the taste buds were jacked up on cookies, ice cream, cake, and greasy junk food. The vegetables may taste pretty bland at first, but after a while, you can taste every nuance of them and savor every subtle flavor. The occasional taste of sugary junk food actually becomes unpleasant. When drama did occasionally make a brief appearance after that, it was quite distasteful, and I recoiled quickly, thanking God for the rich, savory, wholesome goodness of my new drama-free, no-suffering life.

The End of Seeking

YET ANOTHER VEIL was lifted during those long weeks in the silence, and at first it too revealed a vast emptiness. So much of my life had been spent seeking—seeking God, seeking answers, trying every modality, that when that seeking was over, as happens to many people, I scarcely knew what to do. My friend Bob once said about his girlfriend, "If she wasn't a seeker, a recovering something-or-other, and a 'survivor' of something, she wouldn't know who she was." It had almost come to that for me too. I identified so much with the search that the end of it was inconceivable. As my small self slowly relaxed and let go over the ensuing months, I realized that seeking is a way for the small self to hold on, to stay in control.

If the small self can perpetuate an incessant search, it can stay in the driver's seat and continue the charade of seeking relief, while it addictively creates more problems to struggle against and more excuses not to arrive. Once the search is over, and the Large Self is driving, the small self has to take a back seat and let go. There is nothing more for it to pretend it's trying to solve.

There is an old story about a seeker who comes unexpectedly to a door in the woods that says, "God lives here. Welcome, come on in." Elated, the seeker walked up to the door and raised his hand to knock, and then thought twice. He sat on the step perplexed. Soon he stood up, turned around, and walked on down the path. He could not give up the addiction of seeking.

I was ready to give it up. Having thoroughly kicked the drama addiction, I was ready for life to be about creating, expanding, playing, enjoying and loving. I began to wake in the mornings with my mind at quietly at peace, with nothing to worry about or solve. I was accustomed to a mind filled with issues and problems clamoring to be solved. I spent a few days in the emptiness, lying on the sofa, barely interested in eating or doing anything except feeling and breathing, which suddenly seemed like brand new discoveries.

And then one day my body wanted to move about and my mind began to generate some newly productive thoughts. Eventually I knew what to do—each day I did what I was guided to do, doing my best at any given moment to get out of the way, and things started to happen, even where there had been stagnation before.

When talking about what I wanted, I had for some time used the metaphor of how birds fly in a flock at high speeds, swooping and turning and whirling, yet wonder of wonders, they never bump into each other or crash. While scuba diving, I'd watched fish in giant schools as big as a house swimming millimeters from each other, but never bumping into each other, turning in unison—separate, but moving as one.

My wish came true. Life began to flow in that easy way much more often. There is a unified field that connects all life, and the invisible force that orchestrates everything guides all beings *that let go and flow with it*. With steadily increasing ease the inspired thoughts, the solutions, the people, and the circumstances would line up to produce the result needed for everyone involved. My only job was to let go and relax, feel good, and let the universe line it all up. There was awareness that I still had a distance to go in my journey to enlightenment, yet I felt complete ease in putting one foot in front of the other without striving or stressing about it.

I didn't "know" more or have any more "answers" than before; I couldn't see farther ahead than about two stepping-stones in front of me. Nevertheless, I walked with a buoyant feeling that everything was not only all right, but perfectly in order.

During that pre-menopausal crash and long dark slump a few years before, I had wondered if I would ever recover my enthusiasm and confidence. Divine Openings renewed me at age fifty-two—and soon had me on fire with inspiration. I could hardly wait to get into action each day. Things unfolded with amazing velocity. Creativity overflowed in new and delightful forms.

Within seven weeks after the twenty-one days of silence, despite starting over from zero, I had a busy life, full of networking, events, parties, speaking engagements and session clients. I gave Divine Openings every chance I got, and in three months I had given them to about three hundred people. I was more active and inspired than I had been in years, and sometimes worked tirelessly twelve to sixteen hours a day. It was guided action, inspired action. It felt good. Once it was launched and on a steady course, the work diminished and I had lots of playtime. To everything there is a season.

Emptiness is a powerful, fertile womb.

Adjusting to the New Energies

FOR ABOUT THREE DAYS after coming home from India, I laid on the sofa vibrating, just being, and adjusting to the strange new sensations and perceptions. A friend who lived with me said, "Hey, I don't know what you're thinking or feeling, or what's going on." I looked at him with a glint of mischief in my eye and said, "Here, I'll share the contents of my mind with you." Then I gave him the blankest stare for about thirty seconds. After a few seconds, he got it and laughed—there was absolutely nothing going on in my mind, which explained why I had little interest in talking. *The fresh new pure experience of Life was so rich that talking about it paled.* I rarely talk about "it" now except while teaching. It feels better to experience it than to talk about it.

No matter how astounding, how mind-blowing the elevated states are when we first achieve them, they soon feel quite normal to us. A man commented that I had touched his shoulder in passing behind him at a public event, and that he had felt an electric buzz that made him jump and turn around to see who it was, although in that moment I was feeling quite normal. My vibration felt extraordinary to him by contrast (it's all relative) while it felt ordinary to me. Someone will comment how lit up I am, and I might be feeling rather tired in that moment. I am just used to being lit up and it feels like no big deal. You may feel that electrical buzz as you get plugged into a new "energy download" and then it will soon feel normal to you. Or it may be more subtle and gradual for you.

A student marveled at how, after one session, her endometriosis had cleared up, and for the first time in years, she was not balled up in pain during her menstrual cycle with her brain incapable of thinking. Instead, she is happy and energetic. She has felt more at ease than she has felt in years, and her mind is not making up scary stories of what might happen like it used to do. Her eyes are bright and clear, where before she looked dull and low energy.

When I seemed to take it all in stride, she leaned forward and beamed, "This is amazing. This is a miracle!" Then I started laughing. I said, "I know that incredible as all of this is to you, it happens so often now that I think it's just normal! I do appreciate it and thank The Divine every day, but it is no longer so surprising." I was glad she had made such a point of it; it gave me a new chance to see it afresh and rave about it.

Humans "habituate" to things, whether it is ecstasy or pain, and no matter how intense a sensation is, if it continues, it eventually feels normal. You've experienced this with a big new purchase that you've wanted for a long time. At first it seems so exciting to own that new computer with all the fancy features. You gaze at it in awe. "Wow, I can't believe I got this." Within a month or so it seems like no big deal. Sometimes I literally vibrate with newly downloaded frequencies—then I get used to it. As you unfold it is a the increasing alignment with your Large Self that you're feeling, after all.

As your enlightenment unfolds, you will quickly become accustomed to each of the wondrous higher states, and it soon feels just normal. All feelings pass and more will come. Feel the wonder and let it go. There will be another peak.

The ecstatic peak states you may experience at some times are not states our bodies are currently designed to sustain all of the time. While they've wonderful, it's best to enjoy them and let them go. Don't get attached to anything. There can also be a small-self tendency to want the old familiar lows back. The small self is afraid of its own light! Just soften around whatever you're feeling.

The regularly downloaded energy is intense at times because I'm running enough energy to help others as well as expand myself. Sometimes it used to feel like pressure, as if I were trying to squeeze more energy through the pipes than their diameter would allow. But as my capacity to hold that volume of flow and voltage increased, I could do it more comfortably. When I feel the energy increasing now, as it regularly does, I know more is trying to come through. If my small self is resisting and tense—I know to breathe for pleasure, take a hot bath, exercise, or do something that feels good and softens me. Now I know how to let go and let it flow. We must let ourselves keep expanding, because the entire universe is expanding. Resisting hurts—it's supposed to so you'll seek relief!

Creation moves and flows. It didn't stop with the dinosaurs and it won't stop with us. We will never stop moving even after we've achieved a huge degree of enlightenment. We won't seek in that old lackful way, but we will desire, elevate, create, evolve, move, and expand, just as the universe does.

Faster Isn't Always Better

ALL DIVINE OPENINGS except Mother Divine hugs have an "evolution accelerating" effect, so accelerate only as fast as you can release resistance. In other words, when you practice Divine Openings, but then resist feeling, letting go, change, and movement in your life, that's like having one foot on the accelerator and one foot on the brake—so first, release resistance with Divine Mother hugs, prostrating, or some means before you receive more Divine Openings. Move steadily, but ease up on the need for speed. Having high energy plus high resistance burns up your brakes and your transmission.

In practical terms, this means if you're too energized, but not moving forward productively, you need to release resistance, not amp up more energy. If life gets chaotic, slow down, and get grounded with mundane physical things like gardening, walking, cleaning, and organizing.

While reading of the book, you might skip the formal Divine Openings until you relax, let go, and catch up with the acceleration you already have going. Have more fun, and make sure Divine Openings hasn't become work. When you love your life, it doesn't matter how fast it goes—you are free. Racing toward something all the time is pointless unless your life is happy.

Feelings need time to be felt. You cannot feel as deeply when you're running fast, whether it's running toward goals or running away from something. The slower you go, the more you feel. One week I was forced to slow down and do absolutely nothing. It was a revelation. I went even deeper into The Presence. I thought I was already tapped in, but I felt more, much more. Want to get higher and feel more free? Stop running so fast and slow down so you can be more present. You might think you can't afford to slow down, *but you can't afford not to.*

Eventually, you'll stop receiving formal Divine Openings except when you feel called occasionally to get one. Once you can tap in very powerfully on your own, the formal process of receiving a Divine Opening is not necessary. You'll *be* your Large Self, which is the intended result of Divine Openings. At some point everything falls away and there is just the awakened you, with nothing more to "do" except let the expansion continue, enjoy, and live.

As much as I'm committed to everyone becoming inner guided, over the years I've observed that some people want a teacher and some structure for the long run, and that too is a valid choice, just like I'll always continue to rely on my webmaster and accountant for the expertise I won't take the time and focus to master. My specialty in this life is bringing in new energies and guiding people higher. Do what feels right for you. I'm here if you need me, and I'm happy if you don't.

The new energies may feel unfamiliar at first, then will feel normal to you.

The Present Moment Takes Hold

IT BECAME INCREASINGLY hard to dwell on the past or the future as the present became rich and fully captivating. Friends and I would laugh so hard our stomachs cramped, and then the next day not be able to remember what we were laughing about, and it didn't seem to matter. We knew that equally funny, if not funnier things would occur tomorrow. And they did. There was less hanging on to anything. Losses were forgotten just as quickly.

Yes, a few people may accuse you of not caring. They won't understand that suffering over losses, setbacks, or insults is simply a symptom of disconnection from your Large Self. There is truly no such thing as loss from Large Self perspective, but even if you have some temporary sense of loss, your Large Self will find a way to fill in the gap if you allow it. One "downside"? When you live in the moment, if you're not aligned with your Large Self in that moment, it will feel bad. It's supposed to feel bad. It may feel as if this moment will never end—as if this moment is all there is. Because this moment, the eternal now, *IS all there is.*

The Divine is always offering blessings in every moment, and as soon as we let go of the grip on the past, we have an open hand to extend to accept the next gift. Singer-songwriter, turned author, turned 2006 Texas gubernatorial candidate Kinky Friedman says it the down-home Texas way:

When the horse dies, get off.

The Power of Humor

KINKY'S QUOTE IS a good segue way into the next topic: humor. Humor has been a most cherished element of my life for some years now. I already shared with you about creating my own concept of God, and told you that God began to play with me more, and make me laugh. We are most of us far too serious about life, and our early images of God were not funny! They were often serious, unfriendly, judgmental—even scary, vindictive and mean. Little did we know back then that those were the mortal qualities of the humans that created that image of God, not of God Itself.

Long before Divine Openings I set a "serious intention" to have more humor in my life. Each time I've asked for this, Life has turned up the laugh track accordingly. Funny friends showed up, funny movies, funny incidents, funny thoughts and scenarios appeared in my mind for my own entertainment. To this day I am unabashedly goofy with friends and in courses.

I transformed my relationship with my worrying, unhappy, and used-to-be-critical mother by setting a clear intention that every time I called her I would make her laugh right off the starting line. I couldn't change her life, but I could impact my relationship with her and make it a highlight in her day. I collected jokes to tell her, and started our phone calls talking in funny voices, like, "Hello Mommy, did you think leaving me at the mall in 1965 would get you off the hook forever? I know where you live!" Or I'd scream "Mommy! Mooooommmmmy!" into her answering machine, and she'd hear me and run laughing to pick up the phone. For some reason calling her Mommy makes her feel good. Brings back her younger days. Everyone just wants to feel better.

When I first started Divine Openings, Mom sat me down and asked me if I was in a cult. I looked at her with horror and retorted, "I can't *believe* you could even *think* I could be such a sheep! I am *not* in a cult—(I paused for comic effect)—I am *leading* a cult!" She nearly fell down laughing and never brought it up again. By the way, cults separate you from your family and dictate dogmatic beliefs; Divine Openings brings you closer to your family and you choose your own beliefs.

Even when my dad was in the hospital a lot, I'd call Mom and make her laugh. By then she understood (well, at least intellectually) the concept of how important it is to keep your vibration up and she only occasionally gave me grief for not being in grief with her!

Most delightfully, my spiritual power has taken a big step forward each time I asked for more humor. Of course, knowing that everything is vibrational, that's no surprise; humor raises your frequency. I've always gravitated to spiritual teachers with a sense of humor, and avoided the dour, pious, over-serious ones. Ugh, if that's what you get from them, I'll pass. Funny stories in my humor book, *Confessions of a Cowgirl Guru,* will lighten you up as it opens your humor channels up!

Some years ago I was madly in love with a man who didn't laugh much and didn't get my humor at all. I asked for humor in all my relationships after that, and got it. I wrote about it in my first book, *Dating To Change Your Life.* The next relationship was with a man who was very funny, loved to laugh, totally "got" my humor, and thought I was the funniest person he'd ever met. We laughed daily and had a smooth, carefree, harmonious domestic life that was perfect for that stage of our lives, though not a match on the romantic level. There was eventually a parting, and we moved on to more fulfilling partners. I never again dated anyone who didn't have a well-developed, light, and enthusiastic sense of humor.

A former romantic partner of mine turned an interview with 2006 Texas gubernatorial candidate Kinky Friedman into a friendship. Kinky is funny as hell but completely deadpan, and is used to being the funny one himself. After observing the man and me together for a bit Kinky inquired, "Is this a serious relationship?" Without missing a beat, I offered, "No, this is a humorous relationship."

That relationship was marked by frequent laughter, and often, it was out of control, wheezing, snorting, belly-aching, side-splitting, donkey-braying laughter. We looked for opportunities to make each other laugh. One day he had just had a Divine Opening and was in my living room standing on his head doing his karate workout, when he saw the dog's tail bouncing by outside the window. From his upside down viewpoint he thought it was some kind of strange bird hopping by on one wing. He got so broken up when he realized it was the dog's tail that he toppled off his headstand and couldn't get up for laughing.

It's always my intention to look for reasons to laugh, but just as often, reasons to laugh find me. That same friend was poking around checking where he'd left his glasses. He lifted the sleeping dog's butt up and looked under it. Now, I don't know about you, but I had never seen anyone look under a dog's butt for a lost item, and I ripped into convulsions of stomach-cramping giggles, which invariably leads to wheezing, which got us both going even more. Before long, we were both paralyzed and gasping for breath.

Another time, he made a really good omelet with vegetables and avocado. Doing omelets properly had always escaped me. I sleepily said I'd cook next time if he'd "show me how to cook one of those, uh, folded-over things." We were off, laughing uncontrollably, the sounds of our hooting cracking me up even more. I snorted with food in my mouth, then grabbed a napkin to prevent food-spraying, upon which he said, "If you don't watch out, some of that yellow folded stuff with the green filling is going to come out your nose."

So to demonstrate expertly how that could easily be prevented, I stuck the two corners of my napkin up my nose. Then we had a running gag going, and when my long blond hair was in the waffle syrup, he'd say, "Oh, your long yellow stuff is in the sticky stuff." One day he offered, "Here, the feathery red critters made you one of those brown oval things." To that I offered, "There'd be more of those if the long scaly thing wasn't eating them."

When you regain the innocence of a child, there is nothing too silly to do if it will get a laugh, so be generous with your laughter. I remember reading somewhere that polite European society used to deem it unrefined to laugh out loud, and so they suppressed their laughter, allowing only a slight smirk to betray their amusement, lest they look like commoners. There are remnants of that old belief hanging around today, and I am so glad to be free to laugh and show my appreciation and delight. I used to notice in my corporate classes that when people let go of their reserved professionalism and laughed, they really "got" the material and were more alert, happy, and engaged all day.

With very little provocation, just from glancing over and seeing a glint in a friend's eye or a hint of a mischievous smile on the other's lips, I might let go to uncontrollable spasms of laughter. In my retreats, laughter and joy may overtake us for absolutely no reason; it's called "causeless bliss," and it comes from being in the high vibrations of joy and bliss, where laughter is completely spontaneous and needs no reason to be. When you're One with The Divine, there is pure joy of being, and when you live close to that vibration, it takes very little to put you over the top. In many of those moments I truly have no idea why I am laughing—but it feels so good I don't care.

Occasionally, causeless bliss erupts in the Five-Day Silent Retreat. Someone feels a tickle inside and lets it loose, and we all end up hooting like monkeys. You could call it "The Divine laughing you." Tears will come that suddenly turn to bliss. I feel no need to know why. The need to know the why's in life fade the more one enjoys living.

Life may be terminal, but it's certainly not that serious.

As you become your Divine Self more of the time it will even be easier to stop as a disagreement begins and inject humor. Humor dissolves anger and aggravation like nothing else. A partner got angry with me when he was already upset about a work issue, and became defensive at something I said. It undoubtedly activated something very old. I saw the fire flash in his eyes as he set his jaw preparing to fight. Something within me twinkled, and I grabbed his shoulders and looked him straight in the eye, and said, "ME FRIEND!" He was startled at first, and then visibly let go. Then we laughed.

When people get caught up in an emotion, especially an old, chronic, long-practiced one, logic goes out the window. It's as if a lit match was tossed into a dry haystack. Talking about it logically can go in circles for hours, because it isn't logical. You know this. Humor can fire-hose the whole flame in a few words.

Every day brings opportunities to laugh if you notice them. Just start reading funny books, watching funny movies, seeking out funny friends. Remember and tell jokes off the Internet, all the while noticing what it is that makes things funny. Note how funny people, and good story and joke tellers, time their punch lines. There's an art to it and you can pick it up; be easy about it. This isn't work, this is joyful play, and there is no deadline. Pattern your delivery after the pros at first, and then you'll develop your own style. Notice the voice tones they use, and how they play the surprise element to get the laugh. Experiment with how long to pause before delivering the zinger, and pay attention to the things other people find funny. The more you laugh, the more Life will match you up with opportunities to laugh, and make others laugh.

So, what a homework assignment this is! To practice laughter and be funnier than ever before! Write this intention in your notebook, and jot down a few ideas for how to have more humor in your life. If you're an online course member, you could ask for humor inspiration and have fun on the Member Forum.

You can laugh more now.

One night as I lay in my bed giving a long distance Divine Opening to my very ill dad, glee bubbled through me from out of nowhere, and I began to chuckle, then to laugh out loud as I felt his spirit soar. It was a great reminder that no matter how grave the illness, how dire the situation looks from our human perspective, The Divine in us experiences bliss and ecstasy all the time. Knowing this makes any situation better.

A simple way to shift your vibration is to ask,
"What is my Large Self feeling right now?"
The answer is always "bliss" or "all is well."

Divine Opening

THIS WORK OF ART is the pure essence of Grace and joy in uncertain circumstances.

Sit quietly and contemplate the image for two minutes.
Then close your eyes and lie down quietly for fifteen or more minutes.

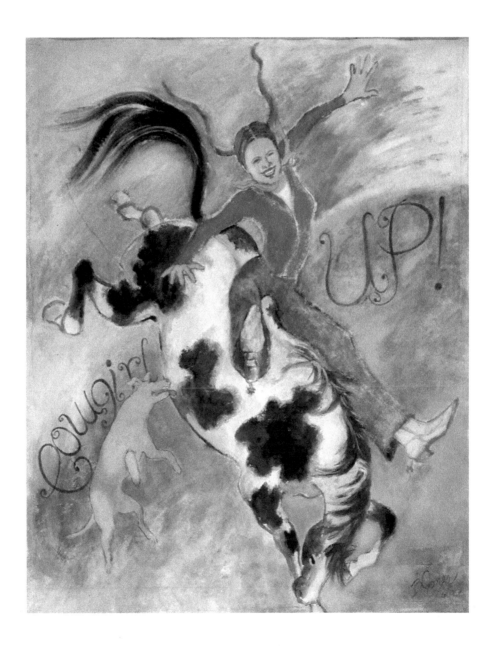

Figure 5 - Cowgirl Up, painting by Lola Jones.

Meditate for Pleasure

MEDITATING GETS EASIER with Divine Openings. Now we meditate because it feels good—not to be good, be spiritual, or get somewhere. Do it to savor your inner silent core and enjoy your expanded self rather than to try to attain some goal. Let go of what other people have told you about their experiences and have your own experience. Deep, sweet feeling is worth as much as all of the mystical visions in the universe. Emptiness is a more powerful state than any vision.

There is no magic formula, and no single way that is best for everyone. I suggest you follow your heart. I keep it very simple. You don't need rules, gadgets, dogmas or complicated secret rituals. If it's too much work, how can you relax and let The Divine do the heavy lifting?

- Sit or lie quietly in any comfortable position. Close your eyes and put a tiny smile on your lips. Focus gently on your breathing. Breathe soft and slow from your belly.

- Now begin to savor your breathing. Notice how wonderful breathing is. Imagine diving down deep into your inner self as you breathe. Think "yes" as you inhale with a tiny smile, and "ah" as you exhale with a slack jaw. You can use those sounds as mantras if you wish.

- If thoughts come, don't "follow them" like a dog chasing a car. Let them go by. Don't fight them. Let them be like voices murmuring in the distant background. Gently return your focus to your breath as many times as you need to without making it wrong that you were distracted. If you get guidance or supportive information, take it, but don't seek it out. When thinking stops, you are out of the way and Grace is in full force. Magic happens in the silence of No-mind.

Meditate for enjoyment, to enjoy the pure essence that is you.

Morning and Evening "Raves"

EACH NIGHT BEFORE BED and when I first woke up, whether I feel great or less than great, I spend a few minutes raving about what I appreciate. Juicy, expressive, and passionate focus on what is good in my life raises my vibration day after day. I routinely celebrate everything I'm happy about to deliberately raise my vibration. Now it's become a natural habit that I practice throughout every day.

Appreciation is the same vibrational frequency as love. Most humans have some highly charged and distorted concepts about love, and may even find "love" hard to muster when they're not happy with someone. But the concept of appreciation is clear, clean, and simple so it's easier to call up appreciation than love. If you can't conjure love for a person right now, you can always authentically find something to appreciate about them.

Raving about what's good trains the mind to look for things to love, admire, and appreciate, then more of those vibrations are magnetized to you. We always have the choice of where to put our focus: on what is "wrong," or what is "right." What is "bad," or what is "good." What we "like," or what we "don't like." Raving has you choose to focus on what feels better. Which feeling or thought brings you more into agreement with your Divine Presence? Does this feel better, or that?

Soon, you find less good/bad duality in your perceptions; it's all considered "experience" and it's easier to soften around "what is" and feel good in any circumstance. Right now you can choose where to put your focus and feel better in minutes. Today is all that really counts. Yesterday is gone, and tomorrow isn't here yet. Right now is where your power is.

In a recent group Divine Opening, as usual I sat with my eyes closed and evoked a powerful vortex for the group of twenty-seven people, and then everyone sat for a few minutes in the Divine Presence and experienced it.

When I asked if a few people would share their experiences, one older woman who was quite experienced on the spiritual path but had struggled with an abusive past shared a profound experience. She saw scenarios from her whole life appear in front of her. Some events had seemed "bad," and others had seemed "good," and they eventually arranged themselves like a mosaic. Then to her surprise she noticed that all of them now seemed equally okay and equally valuable to her. There was no more sense that some had been good and some bad. It wasn't that they all became "good" so much as that it simply didn't make sense to label them anymore. This is the sign of enlightenment called "equanimity" where, by Grace, you inexplicably accept what is or was, without suffering, without story, and without judgment. It's not just a change in perception—*it's a leap to a new dimension of consciousness beyond suffering.*

Another way to define equanimity is softly allowing everything to be as it is, without resisting it. You know it's temporary—everything flows on by—the wanted and the unwanted. And the more freely we let it flow, the more bliss we feel, even in adverse circumstances.

Until appreciation becomes a minute-by-minute habit for you, a morning and evening time of "raving and appreciating" lifts your altitude and your attitude until you naturally reach equanimity, then you are free of the mind and its judgments.

I find it exciting to think that even our wildest dreams of enlightenment and empowerment will pale in the face of what actually comes. We are just beginning to see how we create our reality. In a not-too-distant future, you will literally create worlds, whole realities, for fun. I do.

You can enjoy raving and also allowing what is now.

The Call of the Divine May Sound Like Success, Sex, or Money

MOST PEOPLE AREN'T consciously seeking enlightenment. I used to notice if I mentioned it in a social setting very few people were interested—they were seeking money, a better relationship, freedom from suffering, world peace, better health, clarity, or solutions to problems. These drives for emotional or material desires are fueled by the natural inner drive to feel better, which is the call of The Divine. The Presence within you calls you to feel good and thrive. Although some don't know it, everyone wants enlightenment. They want restoration to their wholeness, which brings bliss as well as the mundane solutions they seek. Whatever they call it, and however they arrive at enlightenment's door is okay with me.

Relationship, health, inner peace, reduced stress, and more money or success are what most people come to me wanting. It's the "big five" that top the list of what most people want and don't have. Their

Large Self lures them home with whatever carrot they most want. One woman had already opened up tremendously by her second session with me. Her mind had quieted, and the bouts of anxiety and worry faded or were short-lived. Anger at her kids had calmed.

Her third Divine Openings session was even more profound. She said she wanted a rich man who would take care of her. "OK, you can have that man," I declared with an authority that comes from The Divine within. "Put it on your list of things you want, and in the meantime I have some things for you to consider."

"First, it's all too easy to start thinking that some person, especially some powerful rich person, is your Source. They are actually just one possible conduit through which Life can send things to you. But what if we get into scarcity, thinking a man is the only place we can get that love or money or care? What if we give our power away to him? Life can bring us what we need through any number of people or circumstances, if we allow it.

"Second, Life brings us more of what we are already feeling. So if you are now feeling a lack of this abundance, and that's why you need this man to take care of you, Law of Attraction can only bring you more lack. If you were to start feeling rich right now, you won't be needy, Law of Attraction can more easily bring you a rich man, you will be a match to his vibration, and so he can stay with you. In America we already are rich as any sultan was two hundred years ago if we just stop and rave about that rather than focusing on what we still don't possess.

"Third, your relationship with The Divine will be reflected outwardly in your romantic relationship. Just for this week, have a love affair with God first. Go directly to Pure Source for the love, the conversation, and the companionship you want—and over time, watch who shows up on the outside. Walk and talk with your Creator, who adores you, loves you exactly as you are, and takes care of you—and can you just imagine who would show up to match that in the physical?"

I evoked a Divine Opening at the end, and went back to my office to write while she rested. After a long rest, tears filled her eyes, and she had difficulty talking without breaking up. She said, "I felt enveloped, hugged, nurtured by The Divine, and then I could feel its Presence sitting next to me, as if waiting to listen, talk to me, whatever I needed. It has filled my empty heart." In that moment, she had moved from lack to fullness.

"Give yourself appreciation for being open to let this gift in," I smiled. "You have opened the door to letting in all good things." That relationship continued to deepen. In the following week, she had some intense neck pain (probably tension or struggle energy letting go), and her chiropractor's efforts to adjust it didn't help. During sleep that night she saw and felt a physical hand press on her neck, and in the morning the pain was gone. I cannot imagine a better example of how our worldly desires for relationship, material things, health, or relief, are always ultimately calling us back to our relationship with The Presence.

Your Large Self is always calling you home in whatever way you are most easily enticed.
You may answer that call now.

How The Presence Sees Us

ONE OF MY EARLY STUDENTS HAD a remarkable experience from her first Divine Opening that continued to unfold for her over many months. She sat perched on the sofa in a room with about twelve people. As I evoked the Divine Opening, she immediately saw herself with nine-foot tall white wings. The most remarkable part of her experience was that she saw herself exactly as The Divine sees her, as absolute perfection. She felt it deep in her being. She'd been an exotic dancer once, and had some self-judgment and doubts about her worthiness. Now there was *no* doubt. She was The Divine looking at The Divine, and it was One with her as she saw every line on her fifty-year-old face in 3-D, lovingly magnified. There was adoration in the gaze. The Presence adores us—it makes no difference what we've done or left undone, no matter who we are or how flawed we believe ourselves to be. Only humans judge. The Divine never does.

Sometimes it's more of a feeling after a Divine Opening, an overwhelming love encompasses you, and in that moment you know you are loved. Sometimes you feel nothing at all, but good things just happen afterward.

Divine Presence adores you . . . because it created you.

Unhooking From Ancient Mind

CARL JUNG SPOKE often of the collective unconsciousness of humanity. Since every thought that has ever been thought is still there, there is a giant pool of collectively shared human vibration you could call Ancient Mind. It is helpful to know that we are much of the time hypnotized by the thoughts and vibrations that we pick up from Ancient Mind, and we buy into a consensus reality that's quite limiting.

The Ancient Mind has long held all but a few enlightened beings in a drama of survival and lack—stuck in suffering, disempowerment and separation from the flow of Life. It's humanity's Ancient Mind conditioning that keeps us tense and resistant. Remembering that the Ancient Mind can hold others hostage helps me feel compassion for people who are doing horrendous things, because I know that they are not at this time able to access their Large self.

Ancient Mind radiates strong vibrations in the range of fear, scarcity, protection, anger, unworthiness, separation and illusion, but also more subtle ones like anxiety or overwhelm, and even positive emotions of joy, love and peace. Until we are highly conscious and awake, we have little choice as to which vibrations we are picking up from it and acting out. Some empathic people pick up stray vibrations far too easily.

Have you ever had a situation where you knew how you wanted to be and act, but couldn't for the life of you do it? We all have. It's like being sucked down into quicksand—wanting to do one thing but to our horror doing something we don't want to do instead. It's as if we've all been plugged into a circuit that charges us up with a discordant energy. When you plug a lamp into the wall, it has no choice about where to get its power. Now we're beginning to plug into a cleaner, purer power source, and the energy we charge up with is different.

I know how impossible it was for me to unhook from it before Divine Openings shifted my consciousness away from it en masse. Divine Openings unhooks us from Ancient Mind, we plug into pure positive energy, and we begin to vibrate more in harmony with Pure Source. There would be no way to "process: all our Ancient Mind conditioning, even in many lifetimes.

Let Grace help you. Just be willing.

As we unhook from Ancient Mind, we sometimes experience the dying gasps of its long-practiced patterns. No worries—they're temporary and they pass, leaving you freer than ever each time. As you activate the higher vibrations, the lower ones die off from lack of attention. Literally, as more humans unplug from Ancient Mind, it loses its power. To set our relationships right we must unhook from Ancient Mind, while having compassion for those who are still in its grip. Not just reading but *doing* the upcoming activities in this book frees you from that conditioning.

The Divine Intelligence waking up within each of us is powerful pure consciousness with no limiting consensus reality. We are the many that are One. We came here to experience individuality, and know our oneness—to create individual realities, but not necessarily conformity.

Ancient Mind is cruel and tells us we are unworthy. Of all the people in the world to set your relationship right with, you are your number one relationship, so appreciate and validate yourself generously. Appreciation is the vibrational equivalent of love, and while we may not know how to "love ourselves more," we can always find tangible things to *appreciate* about ourselves or another.

Every time I do something a little better than before, or any tiny little thing goes well, I hit my "Easy" button. It's a red button from Staples Office Supply. When I hit it, a cheerful man's voice says, "That was easy." By celebrating and appreciating every single thing, I create more to appreciate.

Appreciation is a magical act. Make a habit of giving yourself generous credit, plus some for good measure. Express your appreciation to yourself, everyone, and everything. Appreciation is an important part of the 10% that's yours to do. If you were raised not to build yourself up, how's that been working out for you? If it's hard at first, adore The Presence within you—that's an easy way to start.

Between Worlds

WE STRADDLE TWO dimensions—the old reality in which you have to control your thoughts, and this new dimension where the mind becomes your friend. In the old world we had to work hard to force enlightened thought because our brains were not wired to sustain it. Now Divine Openings literally plugs us into our Larger Intelligence, activates our higher capacities, and upgrades our systems so that we can run "enlightenment software." It replaces the buggy old Ancient Mind software.

When we're no longer slaves to our thoughts and feelings, nor unduly identified with them, it's easier to stay up, or bounce when we dip. Use your Free Will choices minute by minute. At first you'll find you wobble a bit. One day there's peace and oneness, the next day extreme separation as old vibrations activate and move up. One day you may be blissed out, the next you may be depressed. There is really nothing for you to do except "softly embrace your experience." It's all temporary and moves quickly. The day you fear no feeling you are free.

Allow yourself to wobble till you stabilize. Be soft about it.

Your Friend, Contrast

AWAKENED BEINGS still experience contrasts of wanted and unwanted experiences, but tend to use the unwanted experiences as fuel to propel them in positive directions with increased velocity. We bounce off of the unwanted things like we bounce a cue ball off the side of a pool table to sink the bank shot.

Think of contrast as a friend that gives you valuable messages: "Look for a new possibility… get back in the flow… get more in alignment with your Large Self in that area of your life…. here's a place you can evolve." Contrast pushes you when you've held back from moving voluntarily. Contrast challenges you to stretch beyond your old habitual thinking.

When you're cold, contrast tells you to put your coat on. When you don't like something, contrast nudges you to try a new perspective, shift your attitude, raise your vibration, and finally, take inspired action.

Don't just put up with contrast, appreciate it and get in the habit of *looking for the hidden treasure* in it the minute it occurs. Some of my greatest breakthroughs were born of contrast. A retreat was coming up and registration was low because I'd been too busy moving house to get the word out. That contrast stimulated an idea I'd have never have thought of otherwise, and it changed the retreats forever. I sent out a newsletter offering returning retreaters a lower tuition, and many accepted. Those bright beings' presence contributed so much, and made it so much easier for me that I never wanted to have another retreat without them—the lower tuition became standard for returners.

Be willing to fall in love with contrast because even it leads you to new and wonderful breakthroughs. Perfectionistic expectations of never having another challenge, or never again feeling bad only set you up for disappointment. As long as you're human, there will be contrasts, some things you like less than others. Rave about your joys and blessings, and appreciate all contrasts.

As you evolve, as you become accustomed to feeling good, you are going to become *more acutely aware* of the slightest dip into contrast. Don't let your wrong-seeking-missile mind judge that you're slipping backward—you're not—it's just contrast.

Make the most of the best and the least of the worst,
because you create more of what you focus upon.

Let's say ten is the highest altitude possible, and in general, your old set point averaged a five, and you were accustomed to that. Once you start flying higher most of the time, and got used to a seven, feeling a contrast in that old five range now feels as awful as a three used to feel. Five is now your "new low" when five used to be your high. It's all relative, by contrast.

One bright, shining student astounded me when she rated every area of her life at least a nine on a scale of one to ten, yet rated her relationship with her boss as an eight. Most people are delighted with eights, but because she was used to nines, the eight felt really low to her! Eights will feel *bad by contrast* to you too when you get used to soaring on nines and tens. Don't let your mind make the contrast wrong—stay open to the benefit it will bring. She raised her vibration on that relationship to a nine and new possibilities opened in her career.

SUMMARY: Contrasts are a valuable prime driver of evolution, so you might as well embrace every contrast and start anticipating the good that will come of it.

Divine Opening

THIS WORK OF ART activates a specific Energy/Light/Intelligence. Many people reported spontaneous physical healings from this particular piece. It is one of my personal favorites; the originals all hang in my home. Sit quietly, and contemplate the image for two minutes. Then close your eyes, lie down, and savor for fifteen minutes or longer.

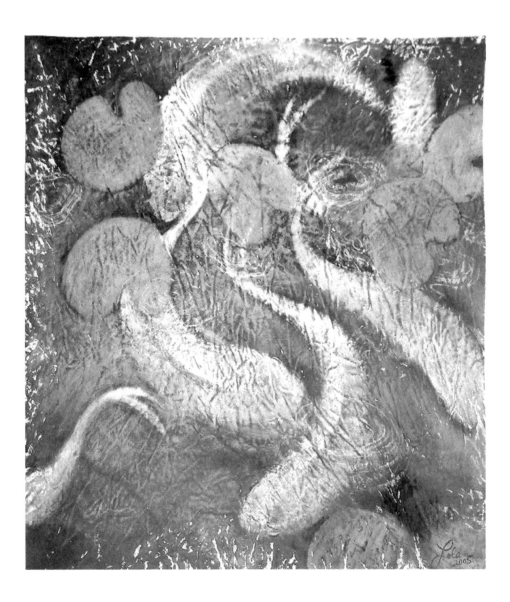

Figure 6—Goldfish, painting by Lola Jones

Romantic Relationships

SO MUCH MAGIC HAPPENS with relationships, I urge you to just witness it with wonder as it unfolds. It's amazing what love feels like when you're free, fulfilled, and in love with life. Oneness with your own Large Self gives security and stability regardless of your romantic life, and who does or doesn't love you. You can experience real love for another person instead of illusion or need. Relationship becomes a whole new experience when your relationship with yourself is already strong and supportive—when there is no emptiness to fill, no lack to escape. The black hole of neediness attracts more lack of love. The painful, aching, longing feeling many people associate with love is actually the feeling of the absence of love or the awful fear of losing it. When you feel full, you attract more love, genuine love. A togetherness that might have seemed excessive or co-dependent in the old paradigm becomes normal and healthy in the new one because it is between two people who know who they are.

Sex is amazing when you feel what your partner is feeling and thrill to it—when you stroke their skin and feel your own pleasure increase. Deeper connectedness in sex goes far beyond physical sensation and friction, and even far beyond love. When love energy circulates in an intimate loop, pleasure increases terrifically, attuning us to our exquisite oneness. When the sense of separation between two people is diminished and they realize they are the male and female counterparts of each other (in heterosexual couples, at least) the intimacy is so sweet. In your partner is a fascinating mirror of yourself. Lovemaking can be a door to higher consciousness when done with love and presence rather than following societal conditioning. Just as there is no ceiling to human evolution, there is no ceiling to love and intimacy.

It's easy to care for another when you know them as yourself and as an expression of The Divine. Fights and conflicts don't happen as often when communication is conscious, direct, and kind. When you know that the other is "You," you cannot hurt them without experiencing pain, just as you can't give pleasure without experiencing it yourself. Relationship problems dissolve quickly when you can be with the emotions that arise and flow through the self and the beloved—when you experience emotion without getting swept up in the story. When you accept others exactly as they are, suffering ceases. When your lover feels your genuine self-generated happiness, the burden is off them to be the source of your happiness. What a relief. Then you can play like children.

I have never, however, insisted that any one romantic relationship must last forever. After two wonderful years, one love and I began to pull in different directions. We were no longer the romantic vibrational match we once were. I felt a deep need to be alone more. I am essentially a free spirit, and found the amount of togetherness he needed stifling. For a while, as friends, we still created together, until he had to stop seeing me so he could move on. Every relationship I've had has been more wonderful than the last.

Relationship for me has been more about spiritual and personal evolution than finding Mr. Right. I have lived so many lives in this body, I can't imagine any one person matching up with all those incarnations of me. It makes most people's heads spin.

Even as I update this book after more than a decade, I only faintly remember the old me who wrote it—my life has expanded so many times. I've lived many new realities and created next level teachings, books, and courses since then.

I love all of my past loves and past selves that were so perfect for that time—real love doesn't end when the relationship changes form. Even if you want to be with someone for life, love lightly, and let it unfold naturally. Let it be however it is. If it's to be for life, it will be. You couldn't possibly stop it.

I did feel that there would eventually be one who could and would fly as high as I wanted to fly, and who would evolve long term with me, on the same, ever-increasingly high wavelength together. I used to joke, "While I don't promise till death do us part, one day that has to happen, because we'll be so old *one of us* will die!" I enjoyed life and happily savored the waiting until he came to me already awake, a powerful creator, my equal, and astounded me with his knowing and wisdom; how he can feel and heal his own body, how he feels me, reads me, opens me, delights me in ways I'd never imagined. He says, "What makes me happiest in the whole world is to see you happy," and he walks that talk.

We live life consciously, deliberately, creatively, and playfully—not perfectly by the way! Along with meditation, tantric sex is a fun part of our spiritual path, opening, expanding, and growing our daily bliss, oneness with each other and with The Presence. If you desire that kind of connection with your current or future partner, that is beyond the scope of this book, but you may enjoy The Art of Love and Sex Online Course (in German and English.)

Unconditional Love: a Practical Definition

EVEN BEFORE DIVINE OPENINGS I never understood how people "stop loving" someone after a divorce, breakup, or disagreement. To stop loving someone is to close our own love pipes, to cut off the flow of our own Life Force. It literally distances us from our unconditionally loving Large Self.

Conditional love says "You must be a certain way to get my love." Unconditional love says, "*I am happy no matter how you are.*" You thought I was going to say "I will love you no matter how you are." No, you don't have to *like* what they do, but when you are happy and being your Large Self *you just love,* because your Large Self *is* love! Real love doesn't go away when the beloved leaves you or changes. If it goes away, it wasn't really love—it was addiction, or a filler for your emptiness, or possession, or entertainment. True love remains, even if you choose not to live with that person, or they choose not to live with you.

This gets easier once the Divine Openings have worked on you for a while. Divine Grace allows us to do in minutes what we've struggled with for years. Grace, that gift we don't have to earn, can do for us what we have not been able to do for ourselves.

Till then, constantly refocus your thoughts on what is good in your partner. What you focus on increases. If you focus on what you appreciate about them, you will get more of that. If you focus on what is wrong with them, you will get more of that. Choose wisely. If you find yourself dwelling on their faults, take a minute or so every day to ponder their good points. Remember how you adored them when you first met? It's the same person after all. Only your focus has changed. The mind, wrong-seeking missile that it is, delights in finding what is wrong. Your Large Self sees only what is right and what good is coming.

The mind is a wrong-seeking missile.
You don't always have to always listen to it!

After receiving Divine Openings for a while, one man was delighted that his thirty year relationship with his wife flowered into happiness again after many stalemated years, as he suddenly became aware he had been passively aggressive while appearing nice and cooperative. The old habit melted away and he experienced pure love for his wife again. As the negativity that is not You rises in vibration, love is what's left.

It is possible that you and your love will become like honeymooners again. Or you may move out of vibrational alignment and evolve in different directions, or one may choose to stay in the same vibration while the other wishes to expand. In that case, you can part with love, blaming no one.

Keep your own love pipes open as you part—if you shut *any* of your love off, your flow is constricted, not theirs. Feel it with acceptance, and stay open. The energy will move, the pain will pass, and with your pipes open and flowing, you're free.

Since there is no sense of scarcity when one is in the flow, relationships of all kinds can move in and out of your life, and you feel no more than a fleeting sense of loss, knowing that you will always have the love you want, both within and outside of you.

Love is endless.

Lay It All Down at the Feet of the Presence

HAVING NEVER CARED for rituals, at first I merely tolerated the ancient Hindu rituals in India. Some were simple, and some were hours long, and needlessly complex, I felt. While I could feel their beauty and power, appreciated the thousands of years and the generations of masters that had left their legacy in these rituals, and especially appreciated the time and passionate energy the monks spent in doing fire ceremonies for us in the oppressive heat, I planned on leaving all that in India and having a more simple and direct relationship with God, sans rituals, back at home. On some level, doing anything that is too complicated feels like giving power away to it. In my heart I knew my relationship with my Inner Source need never be hard or complicated. It is simple and it is right here in any moment—no special rituals or props required.

One ritual did touch me profoundly and stayed with me. Each morning as we began our day, one of the monks sang a chant in a soaring, otherworldly voice; and the arati was performed, a devotional waving of the lighted oil lamp before the altar. It was not the arati that touched me so deeply; it was the prostration at the end of the arati. When prostrating, we laid our bodies face down, stretched out full length on the straw mats, foreheads flat on the floor, with palms together pointing toward the altar. This ritual will be explained for you in greater detail later.

I was unwilling to prostrate to an altar to the guru, as was suggested. Instead, I turned my devotion directly to The Divine Within. The prostration became symbolic of my merging back into Source, of letting go to the flow of life. It was a powerful way to release resistance. During the twenty-one days we prostrated maybe thirty times total, and my body sighed more and more deeply each time my forehead touched the floor. Sometimes I felt some old burden or unnamable heaviness being laid down as I whispered through tears of relief, "Thank you that it isn't my job to figure *this* out anymore." Or, "Thank God I don't have to carry *that* heavy weight anymore, whatever it was."

You may lay all the heaviness down now.

My forehead came to rest on the floor again and again, a cue for my entire body to relax to a degree I had never before experienced. Tensions, burdens, fears, and limitations I had been carrying for God-knows-how-long melted away—no work, no understanding, no processing. Eventually I must have laid it all down; my body relaxed to an astounding extent. This release of resistance showed up in many ways, but one tangible way was that my hips became so flexible and free, and swayed so much when I walked that I felt boneless. My hip never popped again. It was a delight just to feel my body glide along the long gravel road from the dorm to the meditation hall. A body worker asked me after the program how I got so loose; she had never seen anyone walk with such freedom in their hip joints, even after extensive body work. She wanted to know my secret. I told her, "It's release of resistance! It's letting go." Many there unfortunately didn't know how to release their grip of control, to relax the mind's resistance.

Afterwards, at the beach at Mahabalipuram, it was again demonstrated to me just how relaxed and alive my body was. Someone well-recommended offered me a massage for ten dollars American. I looked at him blankly, as if the very idea of needing relaxation did not compute. My head fell back as I smiled a big toothy smile. I could not comprehend wanting a massage. I went for a blissful walk on the beach instead, still smiling at the thought and marveling at the pleasure I felt in my body. After the thirty-two hours of travel home, I was not tired, stiff or jet lagged. My body is still in that relaxed state most of the time now. If it's not, I prostrate and breathe out the tension and resistance! When I lead processes including prostration in my retreats the group energy intensifies the power of it.

Dr. Hans Selye is commonly known as the father of modern stress management, and in the 1950s he demonstrated that the brain of the average normal person operates in a chronic state of survival stress that would be perfectly appropriate in a life-threatening situation, like fighting a lion or running from a bear. Worse, we have become so accustomed to that, we think it is normal. Everyone accepts it. It was only after prostration that I finally knew what a relaxed body could feel like, and that was my new "normal" point. To this day I maintain a much, much lower baseline of stress. I can sit at the computer and get tense shoulders and simply release that tension by intention, a bath, a stretch break. If I want help I get bodywork. And since we can pass along evolutionary advances to others, my students pick this up very quickly. Many completely "lose" their steady state of stress and anxiety at the retreat without working on it at all.

The relaxing of tension was the first of many increasingly pleasurable realizations of just how physical enlightenment is. The more it unfolds, the more I experience it as a full body phenomenon. It's not transcending the body, ascending out of the body, or conquering the body; it is fully inhabiting the body, beyond any sensory experience I've ever had. It's having almost orgasmic ecstasy in mundane moments, finding profound pleasure in simple experiences, laughing or streaming tears of profound bliss for no reason. It's a lightening up of the physical while simultaneously being more grounded. I look forward to hearing how this goes for you.

Prostrating to the Presence

HERE IS A DETAILED "how-to" for prostrating when you want to powerfully and clearly give something over to The Presence. Prostrate for the pure pleasure of it, or to further relax into the supportive arms of The Presence. I don't prostrate in a pious attitude, or in a "please save me" way, or in an "I am unworthy" posture—those are very low vibrations. Prostrating does clearly demonstrate to my small self that I fully intend to let go to my Large Self, to greater ease. Most of all, I do it because it feels so good!

Prostrating can be a physical form of Diving In. Before you prostrate, if your mind is busy, empty it out to your Large Self. State what you need, then drop the story and feel your body. The Presence already knows what you want—prostrating just clearly and physically demonstrates that you're ready to let go of it and let The Divine do the heavy lifting!

Lay down all the big things, the hard things, like releasing hurts, opening your love pipes in relationships, big challenges. Express your intention to let go of being right, working hard, and doing it all yourself. Prostrate to know wisdom, release resistance, get liberation from suffering, meet a challenge, create something new—whatever you want. This ritual helps unhook you from Ancient Mind and become a force for the enlightenment of the planet.

There is nothing magic about any ritual, but rituals like prostrating can help you *focus your energy* in a powerful way. Just don't give the ritual itself your power. Prostrating is a tool to help your mind and body let go. Change the prostrating ritual in any way you desire.

Prostrating Basics:

- Write or speak to yourself about what you want to let go of, put your hand on your heart, or hands in a praying position— whatever feels right for you.

- Sit quietly—feel your full feelings, soften and allow them to be, and drop the story.

- Prostrate on the floor or bed. Lie face down, body stretched out full length, with your forehead on a hard pillow or rolled towel/ Stretch your arms out above and in front of your head with palms together, as in praying position. You can lie on your side or kneel if you prefer.

- Lay it all down. Let go. Stop thinking and trying to solve it, and feel your body.

- Breathe deeply, in big sighs, "for pleasure."

- As you exhale with a whooshing noise, let it all go, intending it all be released to The Presence. Feel the relief when your body gives a final deep sigh.

- Ask to be filled with the feeling and knowing of You as Divine Presence.

Lay down anything and everything that's too big for you.

Sickness and Health

IN THE TWENTY-ONE days of silence, about 80% of the people experienced the dissolution of old patterns, childhood conditioning, and other negativity as *physical sickness* rather than feeling the emotions directly. I didn't experience any sickness because I was guided to be with feelings and move it all emotionally. Those who feared lower emotions, ran from them, stuffed them, or thought it made them less spiritual, tried to do the spiritual bypass and mentally gloss over the lower feelings. It doesn't work.

Back at home, one of my students had repeated accidents as he resisted feelings and avoided claiming he creates it all. In his case, the contrasts demonstrated how he made choices that hurt himself. Physical manifestations are the hard way to discover the lower energies we're vibrating. Accidents are often caused by believing life is random and accidental.

Masses of lower energy move up with Divine Openings. This is rapid, en mass movement, not the never-ending, bit-by-bit, old-paradigm process that takes a long time. Some people let it move without fanfare; with no resistance, and with total ease. If "all hell breaks loose" when you begin Divine Openings, that tells you it was *way overdue*. Think what would have happened if you'd waited longer? The good news is that it passes quickly if you don't make it wrong or resist what's happening. Some move it with emotional discharge, others with physical discharge or sickness, others by seeing it in the mirror of life.

Any movement is always a good sign. The higher you ascend in altitude, the greater the necessity to jettison any density that no longer aligns with you. As that density rises to higher vibrations, it may be effortless, or it may take the form of discomfort, low emotions, or fatigue. Some people actually like intense physical symptoms, because they need a sure sign that something powerful is moving.

We're understandably very concerned about our bodies, and physical diagnoses of dis-ease are some of the hardest things for people to relax into acceptance about. When a doctor is saying you have a dis-ease and shows you a chart with evidence, it takes intention, clarity, and focus to disregard that authoritative proclamation and hold to your desired image of health until your vision overpowers the temporary reality of the disease. Stop giving so much *respect* to any unwanted reality—it's all temporary unless you keep giving it reality.

I rarely like to call out the names of dis-eases, because it tends to give them more reality. Thought, emotion, matter, Spirit—it is all just vibration at different densities. Divine Openings can interrupts it at a high vibrational level, allowing the body to more easily restore itself to balance.

Most of us think we only *observe* reality. But observing it is *creating* it. We observe what is, and vibrate what is, which creates more of what is. Then we observe what is, vibrate what is, and create more of what is. The only reason any reality exists is that you vibrated its essence long enough. For example, when a person vibrates insecurity or concern, stress or anger for long enough, it can eventually manifest as a dis-ease. The well-being that constantly flows keeps you healthy and corrects problems. Lack of flow is the basic root of all dis-ease.

First, soften and accept where you are. Stop observing/creating what is, and turn your powerful attention to what you do want. Then you begin to let in what you want. Then as you observe the improved situation, you let in more improvement. Feel the vibration at its core, be open, let Grace help. Always follow your own guidance foremost, and get any medical help you need in addition. This life offers unlimited possibilities, and modern medicine can be a miracle too.

Do not blame yourself for creating illness. We are human! If you are dealing with physical illness or pain and still cannot get relief, never allow yourself to suffer or be stuck for long! There are no limits to what can be healed or resolved. None. Check the additional resources at the end of this book.

Who Are We?

YOU'RE NOT SOME inferior being here to earn your way to some reward. You're not here to earn your worthiness. You are magnificent—the Divine's finest creation, pioneering expansion in the physical dimension. This wondrous world of tastes, smells, light, sound, and touch needs to be tasted by your lips, smelled by your nose, and seen with your eyes. Life enjoys living through us, and it's our choice whether we enjoy it or not! There is great celebration in the Non-Physical realms when we do.

For millennia, Life has evolved us as a species, developing and preparing our minds and bodies to embody more of The Presence. But new energies coming to the planet now are catalyzing quantum leaps for us by pure Grace, as we prepare for the full descent of Spirit into matter (or you could see it as matter ascending into light.) You may call the awakening whatever you like; the Mystery cannot be explained by the mind, but it can easily be enjoyed.

The Grace that Divine Openings opens you to gives the brain increasing capability to sustain the higher states and directly experience reality so that we can walk the Earth knowing ourselves as aspects of God. Our physical bodies are evolving to fully embody it long-term.

The Essence Of Life always remains in its vast, formless, multi-dimensional, timeless, Non-Physical state, but it focuses aspects of itself into many physical forms, including beings like us. Our bodies and the physical things we create are fleeting manifestations, but our Essence continues on through it all, evolving in Intelligence and Wisdom backwards and forwards in time.

There's no risk for an eternal being, since there is no death; there is only life and more life. It was such a freedom when a near death experience showed me I really was not afraid to die! I was actually debating, "Go? Or stay?" with no attachment to the outcome. Now I can always find that still, unshakable center inside me that is always steady, no matter what is happening outside. All I do now is tune in, and get myself to the party. Anytime you stop and be still you can find it. Set aside time every day to tune in, whether in meditation, moments of silence, or nature walks.

It became increasingly clear it was always there inside anytime I wanted to experience it. I'd known this as a mental concept for years, but now it was vividly real. Adventures await you on this Earth and within, and your capacities continue to increase astoundingly. You're just beginning to tap in, and the more you do, the more you discover your unused gifts and capacities.

While it may not always be obvious from our small-self perspective, from Larger perspective, we are the early astronauts, braving the unknown to satisfy an inexplicable need to expand our world beyond the prescribed limitations of the old order. Like their Command Central Ground Control, our Universal Intelligence acts as a navigational base system for us, giving us all the support we need to do anything successfully. Our job is to keep our vibration high enough to receive and interpret it accurately, sort of like keeping our satellite dish pointed toward that steady home signal rather than pointing away at worthless, discordant distractions. We're evolving away from the judgment and the suffering caused by the mind's domination. We don't have to know how to do it. Our desire sends out a call, our Large Selves births solutions and deliver them as vibrational signals, we interpret them, and we take steps as guided.

It is, after all, our physical selves that expand the physical world, by experimenting in the duality and contrast of the wanted and the unwanted, the "good" and the "bad," while the Essence Of Life remains reliable, blissful, and non-dual. Remember, when you're feeling strong desire for something that isn't manifested yet, it's there for you. If you vibrate in harmony with that desire, you get to experience the joy of it right now, and then it's a bonus that as you vibrate it consistently, something materializes to match it. Even if you don't manage to see it happen in your lifetime, you created it, and contributed it to the evolution of this and all other dimensions. Imagine those science fiction writers like Jules Verne who didn't get to see their stories become reality in this lifetime—they get to experience it in the next. Your desire is never lost or wasted, but waits for you in some other body, place, or time. What we'll evolve into next is beyond imagination. You'll take with you all of your expansion, and go beyond even that. Just imagine it, for fun.

Leading the Universe's Expansion

THE CREATOR HASN'T laid out a plan for all eternity. Creation is ever new, always experimental, always expanding. There's no master plan all finished, waiting for us to figure it out and get it right. There's no test to pass, no wings to earn, no cut to make. There is nowhere to get to because there is no finish line, but you get to do with this life whatever you choose. You are free.

The universe is one eternal, ecstatic explosion of creativity, and we reflect its thirst for experience with more than six billion faces. If you're reading this, chances are that you are one who doesn't follow the norm; you create new possibilities. You're not interested in the status quo. You understand it's all in Divine Order and there's never anything "wrong," but you always want more and better. We're not the cosmic couch potatoes, we're members of a Divine scouting party out on the leading edge of endless creation. Like all explorers, on some level we liked the idea that we'd come to this far-flung frontier where we'd blaze new trails, take risks, try new things, sometimes fail, to get up and try again. You're going to do great things, lightly, easily, breezily.

Ever wonder why you sometimes don't get clear guidance about what to do? It's because you as Divine Presence in a physical body get to create your own directions, inspired ideas, and solutions. You get to try new things, and it doesn't really matter how it works out. There's really no risk in the end because there is no end. You can't fail because it's never over. Of course you want to succeed at endeavors, but soothing yourself this way can help you lighten up and go for it. What do you have to lose? There is guidance, there is that stable base station that has the broader view, with its radar, navigating devices and powerful resources to help, but on this frontier there is no map, only historical evidence, which we're not interested in anyway. We don't want to repeat history; we have bigger desires. Even if it's safer, it's not satisfying. We will continue our exploration of the far fringes of possibility for all eternity, and some of us will come back again and again to this fascinating and yet maddeningly dense and slow (compared to the lightning speed of the Non-Physical planes) physical environment, into the uncertainty of leading edge pioneering.

The Creator is not complete, finished, and perfect waiting for us "defective ones" to get it right, redeem ourselves, cleanse ourselves, or be good so we get rewarded. We are the Creator's adored physical extensions, bringing this physical dimension more into alignment with the spiritual dimensions, just by being joyful, loving, and creative. Isn't it a relief that it isn't work? Heaven on Earth was here all along; it just takes awakened eyes to see it.

Heaven is right here on Earth.

What is Enlightenment?

ENLIGHTENMENT IS NO big deal. It is simply the natural state you were designed to live in. We are meant to be happy, healthy, loving, expanding creatures. When you are living in that state it will just feel normal. Granted, when you first feel the full surge of Life Force flowing through you, it may feel like you've stuck your toe in a light socket. But when you get accustomed to it, it will feel like no big deal. It is your natural state. A magnificent, healthy, vital racehorse feels good in its body, and it is a miracle to watch, but it is not supernatural. *It is natural.*

If you expect something supernatural, you may be disappointed if that's not your Large Self's path for you. Sometimes it doesn't happen immediately but it opens up over time. Sometimes people who did not ask for supernatural manifestations get them! Let The Presence decide. Can you let go and enjoy whatever wonderful gifts come? If so, they come faster.

Before we talk about what enlightenment is, I encourage you to relax about the timing and details. You may or may not experience the "classical" enlightenment. Yours will be unique. As enlightenment flowers, you begin to see, feel and experience things that were there all along, but you were unable to see them, tune into them. Love for an estranged parent or ex-spouse, a personal relationship with The Presence, appreciation for the beauty in everything—these things were there all along. By Grace, a change inside you suddenly makes it possible to perceive subtleties you couldn't before—mysteriously your AM radio is replaced with an FM radio and now you can get those stations that existed all along, but simply did not exist on your old AM radio dial.

You are literally being hooked up to a rich, complex world wide web, and you don't have to know how it works to enjoy the miracle of it. You don't have to know how a computer works, what makes your heart beat, or how the plants you eat grow to appreciate and benefit from them. As you rediscover your oneness with the unified field, you are once again in harmony with The Essence Of Life that orchestrates everything. When you live consciously as your Large Self, you are led where you need to be; synchronicity has you rendezvous easily with the perfect people for mutual benefit and mutual joy. You know that well-being enfolds you.

Divine Openings causes a moment of birth—there's a crossing of a threshold into enlightenment, and yet it is never quite "finished." The entire universe is expanding, and so are we. If you ask an enlightened being, "Are you enlightened?" the answer is something to the effect of, "I am still evolving, just as everything is still evolving, expanding, and becoming." One who is enlightened has no need to say so. One who has a need to say so is not yet enlightened.

For some, the flowering of enlightenment begins to happen within a few days of their first Divine Opening. For most it is a gradual unfolding and savoring of each new step as they acclimate to a wholly new world. My own process was more gradual, unfolding over years, and it is still deepening. I feel The

Divine gave me a more gradual process so that I could remain in a normal life, relate easily with regular people, and they can relate to me in my imperfection. I help soothe the fears of their small selves, and help them release resistance from a place of having been through it all myself, rather than receiving it in one flash of illumination. The big cosmic flashes aren't always the silver bullets you might imagine them to be.

Slow down and savor each day! Slower is often faster.

We are Life Energy in human form, playing in creation. When I first saw who I really am, my small self was afraid of the light of my own Being. Your mind may continue to deny that enlightenment has begun to flower and try to continue its old routine. A fan continues to turn even after you turn off the switch. It will slow and stop after a while.

As consciousness expands, we gain conscious access to a broader perspective, and that is what I call "being my Large Self." The Large Self is more wise, loving and powerful than the narrowly focused small self. The small self doesn't need to know all the details when it follows the guidance from the Large Self at Command Central. Astronauts don't need to know every instrument reading that NASA is seeing from the ground; they get the information they need in the moment, to get where they want to go, or to do the job at hand. Your small self is the astronaut; your Large Self is Command Central.

The Supreme Creator, spanning many universes, many dimensions, and many realities, with its perspective so broad, so vast that we cannot conceive of it, decided to express a small part of itself as a focal point in you—you are a somewhat narrowed creative focus of Source. The vastly Larger part of you always remains in the Non-Physical realm, but you always have access to its resources. Now you can walk the planet as that Large Self, playing this game we call "life on planet Earth" in full awareness, conscious of that Larger You, awake to all of who you are.

Enlightenment is becoming conscious.

Classic Signs of Enlightenment

YOU WILL BEGIN to experience signs of enlightenment and may wonder what they mean. The earliest signs of enlightenment are usually increased inner peace, a quieter mind, moments of causeless bliss, and mysterious disappearance of anxiety. Synchronicity amps up. Once you relax into the flow of life, its natural orchestration brings people, circumstances and events together to provide what's needed for all. Life is all connected, all intelligent, all one, so of course it works in concert with your needs and desires. Science calls it the unified field.

I asked for a very functional, grounded, connected, practical form of enlightenment, as I wanted to be fully engaged with the world and its business, not to sit in meditation my whole life. Some do want to merely sit and beam enlightened energy to the world from a distance. That's a worthy service—if it's what you want. I wanted a practical, grounded, and fun enlightenment. I wanted it to make me even more effective in my worldly affairs and more loving and available in relationships. You can design your enlightenment just about any way you want to, and later in the book you'll get help doing that.

While there are some classic signs, your enlightenment is unique and not everyone experiences the "classic" variety. These signs may not all appear at once, but as part of an unfolding.

1. Witnessing yourself: Observing yourself objectively from your Large Self is one hallmark of enlightenment. This "witnessing" of yourself may occur as an actual out-of-body experience where you look down upon your body. It may be a more subtle perspective, with your wiser, objective Large Self noticing the actions and responses of your human self with love and discernment, but no judgment. That's how I usually witness. You begin to see the workings of your own mind and emotions rather than being lost "in them." Suddenly you see clearly the old habits and beliefs that have ruled your life. The mind may not entirely stop doing what it does, but it no longer controls you because your awareness is larger than your mind. You begin to understand that you're not your mind. "Just because my mind says something doesn't mean I have to listen!"

You become less and less identified with your small self's dramas, stories and distortions and more identified with your Larger Self view. You don't stop being human and fallible, but you are more conscious, aware of what you are feeling, saying, or doing. You are not run by it. Now I can reach deep states of meditation even when my mind is chattering away. I can witness it and ignore it.

2. Equanimity and the end of suffering: The ability to fully experience each moment as it comes your way, without suffering, is "equanimity." This aspect of enlightenment allows us to experience current physical reality, other people, and our own emotions *as they are*, without resistance to them. We appreciate and accept everything as it is, at peace in the calm in the eye of the hurricane. Experiences move by in a kaleidoscopic parade. There is less story and more pure experience. We often say, "It is what it is," or "How interesting that I created *that*," or "Everything is temporary—this too shall pass." We can be productive no matter how we feel.

Enlightenment has been called the end of suffering. I had a dear friend who was fifty-six, in a nursing home, bedridden, dependent on dialysis, on disability income, and lost both legs from diabetes. I gave him Divine Openings over many months. He went through a deep dark night of the soul at one point, diving to the depths of despair. He left his body and communed with dead relatives in a vast white space with no floor or walls. Then he emerged peaceful and joyful. By the time he passed away, he was one of the happiest people I knew. He uplifted the doctors and nurses. Even though his body was diminished and he could not reverse it at that point, he did not feel powerless.

My personal experience has been a gradual loss of the ability to suffer—literally to the point where very little disturbs my inner peace for longer than a few minutes, or at the very worst, a few hours or a day. When we experience things from Large Self perspective, or God perspective, there is nothing to suffer about. Even if someone dies, we know there is no real death, just a change of form. If we lose something or someone, we know that there is no scarcity. When we look at suffering in the world, we hold the energy of the solution, rather than suffering over their suffering, which only adds to the suffering. You can't work on this—it will come if you simply stay the course.

3. Oneness, or unconditional love: Love is the most important aspect of enlightenment. Psychic powers, manifesting, and mystical visions are trivial, even useless, if love is not flowing. The flowering of the heart deepens enlightenment, bringing the experience of oneness with All That Is. You might suddenly feel causeless love for strangers, or feel like everything is inside of you or that you are indistinguishable from everything. You might talk directly with nature, bring rain, communicate with animals, or somehow know what someone needs. You tap into Universal Intelligence to know useful things in your areas of interest, whether it's science, car repair, or business. There is no longer any sense of separation between you and All That Is. You're aware that you are a distinct part of All That Is. It usually comes in peaks, but you are forever transformed unless you choose to "go back to sleep."

With some things in life, you might want someone to tell you what to expect, give you the benefit of their experience; but you are urged to go into this very personal spiritual adventure *open to discover* the unique gift The Divine has for you. You cannot fail at this, and perfection is not the goal of this ever-expanding universe, nor is it a qualification for enlightenment. There will be more on this topic as the book progresses and as you go through your experience.

Once you've begun the unfolding of enlightenment, it's like being on a plane from New York to California; there's no need to stress about whether you'll get there or not. You can't make the journey go faster by running up and down the aisles, so you might as well relax and enjoy the ride. Each stage has its own sweetness, so enjoy it. You will arrive at the scheduled time!

There are classic signs, but your enlightenment will be unique.

Powers and Mystical Phenomena

POWERS AND MYSTICAL phenomena are wonderful talents and useful gifts, but they are not synonymous with enlightenment. One who can perform impressive feats, give psychic information, heal, see guides or other dimensional beings, but still withholds love from family members or loved ones, or lives in scarcity, conflict or fearfulness, has still not experienced the flowering of enlightenment.

As your enlightenment unfolds, you may be expecting to see or hear certain things that you've heard or read about, such as visions, voices, entities, angels, masters or light phenomena. You may—or you may not. If you'll release all your concepts of what a spiritual or religious experience should be, you'll appreciate and enjoy your own unique experience much more. Comparing, and expecting someone else's experiences to happen to you is a setup for disappointment. No two people's enlightenment will be the same, or look the same, nor should it. Your gifts will be completely unique and your appreciation of them will increase them.

Some will see other dimensions and auras, spiritual entities, angels, or guides. Others will never have any such experience, *and it does not matter! There is no goal.* Personally, I don't experience Source as a separate entity from myself at all. It occurs for me as a direct knowing, a deep empty bliss, or as my Large Self speaking. The more you can experience it fresh, the purer and more distortion-free it will be.

Consider that angels, guides, beings, and even visions of God are all *manifest forms*, while the purest essence of The Creator is *formless*, Non-Physical, and pre-manifest. In the very deepest oneness with The Presence, there is nothing but the silence of The Void. Enlightened singer/composer Miten says in his song, *Empty Heart*, "I tried to name the nameless. I tried hard to understand. When I closed my fist, well of course I missed. There was nothing in my hand. I've got this empty heart, that I can't explain. No longing for love, no sweet pain. No voice I hear in the still of night, just an empty heart, full of light."

I encourage you to clean out all your mental closets of old concepts of what you think spirituality is, and what you think God is, and what you think the point of it all is. If no one had influenced you—if no one had written books about it—what would you experience? Research shows that people experience God as their culture has trained them to. In mystical experiences, Christians see Jesus or Mary or angels. In the ancient East no one ever saw them—they saw Krishna or Ganesha, Mohammed or Buddha. There is little variation within each culture's experience, but there is drastic variation between cultures. That is conditioning, not fresh, authentic experience.

What if you forget what books and culture and other people said, and have a direct, personal experience? You could have your first-ever pure, authentic spiritual experience. People are often so busy chasing something they read about that they miss their own experience!

For many like myself, the deepest experiences are of pure feeling, direct knowing, or the blissful silence of the Void. In my retreat initiations many people do have dramatic and vivid experiences, because the retreats get you so out of the way, but those who have more subtle initiation experiences can have lives that are just as happy. Don't judge or compare—it's all good.

One morning I woke up and felt physically and emotionally bad. So I relaxed into the feeling to experience it fully, so it could move up to a higher vibration. Within ten minutes not only did it move, but I was in such deep bliss that I laid there for another half hour just luxuriating in it. When the bliss body lights up, it feels ecstatic just to breathe. And then you'll get used to it and it will be normal for you. Those experiences are far more common for me than flashy phenomena, and I love them. I would not trade them for anyone's cosmic experiences. They're authentically mine. Have your authentic experience.

What every human being wants is to feel good and be happy, so think about this: why do people so desperately want to hear guides and see angels? To help them feel better! You will soon feel much better, and when you feel good, you won't care whether you ever hear a spirit guide or saw an angel.

Now you can have your own authentic spiritual experience.
It will deepen and expand naturally.

You May Design Your Own Enlightenment

ONE OF MY GREATEST fears about the twenty-one days of silence was that I'd come out of it unable to live in this world, relate to regular people, and deal with the practical day to day aspects of life. Then I realized I could design my enlightenment however I wanted. I had apprehensions about the program. There was too much power given to the gurus, but I didn't give them any of my power—I let in only the part I wanted and left the rest. There is no dogma or rules in Divine Openings, only teachings that you might find empowering and helpful on your journey.

The last fear, the fear of losing my "separate self" or personality, I would have to deal with. Some went there asking for mystical experiences and cosmic consciousness. Some actually wanted their personality to be erased, but enlightened people who have completely erased their minds are sometimes barely functional in the world. That's OK for a monk, esoteric teacher or someone who isn't interested in the material world, but I was clear that I wanted full engagement in this world. The enlightenment I designed and asked The Divine for was a practical one that would have me be effective in life, business, relationships, and all aspects of the material world.

Isn't it funny how we don't completely trust our Large Self, the unlimited part of us, to know what's best for us? We trust our car to start, the sun to come up in the morning, and the airplane to stay aloft, but we don't trust our own Innermost Self! It was weird, knowing that surrender to The Divine was the way to go, but not fully wanting to do it. That's how humanity has gotten in the state it's in, being determined to do it "our way" even if it's the hard way.

If you can let go of any concepts about what enlightenment *is,* an authentic enlightenment unfolds for you. Most of the literary accounts and known examples of enlightenment are of spiritual teachers, but not everyone is meant to be a stereotypical spiritual teacher. Enlightened people are now blissful in high-tech jobs, driving buses, filling prescriptions, and raising children. One of our Certified Guides lights children's minds and spirits up through brilliant math tutoring, and she loves her life.

I see people suffering unnecessarily over their careers, struggling unsuccessfully to be healers or teachers when that is not their path. We need enlightened people in all roles in life, from bakers baking with love, to maids cleaning with intention, to CEO's leading enlightened corporations. So please don't succumb to the popular mania that you would be happier or more fulfilled in some other career that has more spiritual "significance" or prestige.

I had given up teaching, knowing full well that being an artist would be just as good. Then surprisingly, I was called from within to return to teaching. Folks, if you're called to teach or heal, you will not be able to stop yourself! If it doesn't flow for you, pay close attention to what does flow, and do that. You will make a difference for others in any career just by being you, lit up.

Just as in my concept of God, in my enlightenment I wanted to include lots of humor and fun, playfulness and spontaneity. A real cowgirl is not the least bit interested in qualities like saintliness and piety. I wanted only enough gravity to be credible and taken seriously; my gift is more to lighten people up than to be the serious, heavy type—how boring! Each of us is a broadcast tower in our daily lives. We're always beaming something out there whether we're doing business consulting, serving food, or repairing someone's car. Enlightenment makes you a beacon no matter what you're doing. There is no profession unworthy of an enlightened person, or lesser than any other profession. If you enjoy it and are good at it, it's valuable. I'd like to see farming become an enlightened profession, with farmers who are one with the land, plants, animals, and ecosystem, and produce vibrant, healthy food, and a clean environment. One Divine Openings Five-Day Retreat attendee in northern California can direct her cattle around the farm with her mind.

What would you like to include in your enlightenment, and what would you leave out? Spend a few moments getting curious about it. You'll discover new parts of yourself that you cannot now imagine once it begins to unfold. You'll keep revising it forever. Have a little fun daydreaming about it. You are a powerful creator, a miracle worker. What talents do you have and what might you do with them?

APPLY IT TO YOUR LIFE: Write in your journal now or create a vision board. Imagine how you'll feel in your most ideal world, just for fun. Be unattached to specifics and open to unknown possibilities, because we don't always know what's possible or best for us. The Presence will co-create with you to go beyond your limiting ideas. Drop your ideas completely and let it go before you do the next Divine Opening. Take nothing with you—be a clean slate.

Divine Opening

GAZE FOR TWO minutes, then close your eyes, lie down, and let go.

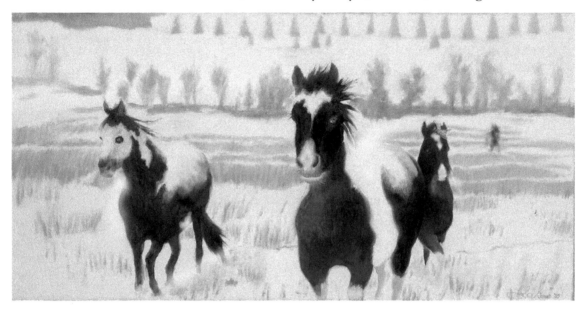

Figure 7—Ghost Horses, *a painting by Lola Jones.*

The art is shown in color in the Art Gallery at DivineOpenings.com if you wish to enjoy it free, but the black and white art works precisely the same.

As many people enjoy this energy in their living and work spaces, printable color art files or large archival prints are available on the site as well.

Negative Manifestations that Still Show Up after You've Raised Your Altitude

FIRST OF ALL, everything that happens is valuable information, and calling it "negative" devalues it. Whatever is playing out for you right now is the perfect product of how you vibrated in the past. It's an echo of your past. If you're not creating that anymore, it's already history, and you can change your tomorrow right now. Appreciate it all and it changes faster.

In this physical world, things that exist in the material today are here simply because energy, thoughts, focus, and feelings (conscious or unconscious) from the past built up to a critical mass to create them. Today's reality is a product of weeks, months or years of that vibration.

Even when you raise your altitude today, some people, events, and things were already in the delivery truck on their way to you. It might (or might not) take a bit of time for the old manifestations to stop being delivered, and for the new things you want to get delivered. You can neutralize any old, pending manifestation right up to that point of momentum where they are already on the physical delivery truck on their way to you.

We think we want instant manifestation, but be grateful that there is a space/time lag before our thoughts manifest. Be glad a particular vibration has to occur consistently for some time before there's enough critical mass for it to show up in the physical. If there wasn't a lag, your slightest fear or worry would show up in front of you within seconds—you'd worry about being eaten by a shark, and presto, a shark, a pit bull, or a lawsuit would jump out and try to chew you up! Fortunately, in this dimension, the time lag allows us plenty of time to catch it and say, "Whoa, better tip the nose up and find a better feeling before something like this manifests!"

NOTE: You don't always manifest literally what you felt or thought about, but the vibration always matches. For example: resisting change and not owning responsibility for our reality attracts broken bones, they snap under the pressure. Feeling like the world isn't safe attracts victimization.

One student started having accidents right after we began our work together. First he sprained his ankle playing with kids. That triggered a worsened dependence on the painkillers and anti-depressants he came to me to get off of. Then the next week he fell down his stairs due to painkillers, and so had to have more painkillers! There are no accidents.

I had an "aha." "Were you always accident prone?" He indeed had an old belief that he was unlucky and life didn't support him—this was just an old vibrational habit. The good news is that with Divine Openings, what comes up is moving up for good. He rapidly got better and went on to kick the addictions that were ruining his marriage. Now he's a new dad, has a great job, marriage and life, and is doing his music again too.

His Large Self knew that there was an opportunity to get it all out on the table and brought him just the "accidents" he needed to see his vibrational habits. He seized the day and took his power back.

Besides feeling good and becoming free of slavery to the emotions and the mind, living in a higher vibration has a stunningly wonderful natural result. The more you live in higher vibration, the better the outer conditions go. If you encounter people and circumstances you are certain do not seem to match, then there is a vibration you are not aware of—I call them blind spots.

The only reason one would not recognize an incident as a natural product of one's own vibration is not being in touch with the feeling or vibration that generated it. Either they have learned to ignore it, numb it, rationalize it, or explain it away—or it has been in their body for so long, perhaps even since birth, that they don't notice or feel it. It's invisible and unconscious.

People become accustomed to a feeling and think it's normal. They have no other experience to compare it to. Unfortunately, we tend to adjust to the pain or lack in our lives, and think of it as normal. An abused child may beg to go back to the abusive parent—it's familiar—it's home.

In other cases, the person is not aware of how important it is to feel good, or they have been brainwashed by a society that doesn't value good feelings. They feel "bad" about choosing to feel good! How sad is that! Do you watch bad-feeling TV and movies, read bad news, and talk about horrible things with no regard for how it makes you feel, and what that creates? If you want something different, change your focus.

Imagine an airline pilot ignoring the altitude reading on his Instrument Panel as the plane heads toward a mountain, or ignoring the low fuel reading until he runs out of gas.

But being conditioned as most of us were, we often did ignore our Instrument Panel. Or the feelings that were amped up by the stories became so painful we had to shut them off. We ran from, resisted, and tried to fix our painful feelings for so long we forgot how to take our own bearings. No one's blaming us for doing that. We just got separated from our own inner wisdom.

 From birth onward, well-meaning people encouraged us to listen to them instead of our own feelings. School in particular was geared to teach us to conform and obey, to listen to outer guidance, not the inner voice, and to tone down our energy, go against our natural desires, and delay the gratification of our passions. So much of what we were taught was designed for the convenience and pleasure of others, not for our empowerment.

So it becomes that we don't know which way is "up" on the Instrument Panel. Some people's Instrument Panel got turned upside down and they thought feeling good was bad, and feeling bad was good. From now on, you'll know which way is up, and you'll come to know that it's simple: *good feels good, and bad feels bad.* There is a whooshing current of energy I feel every time a student catches that tailwind of their Large Self and begins to soar toward alignment with it. "Can you feel that?" I'll ask. Most can. They are remembering how to feel subtle energies they'd long ago become desensitized to. This return to feeling is the door to bliss.

Divine Openings moves feelings and gives you back your energy. Grace does for us what we cannot do for ourselves. Just stick with it and do your part—let go and get out of the way. Choose the highest vibration you can at any given moment. Say yes to every feeling, soften, and life opens new doors to you.

Everyday Relationships are the Key to World Peace

ONENESS WAS MERELY a nice unattainable intellectual concept until I began to have the actual experience of The Divine waking up within me. As the small self lets go, we lose the angst of separateness, competition, danger and scarcity. When we are a part of All That Is, what is there to fear or defend from? We lose our fear of "others" as we realize there are no others. Even though for all practical human purposes I know that my body and my self is separate from yours, I realize we are still part of the same stream of life, we are made of the same stuff, we come from the same Source. I cannot harm the seeming other without literally feeling that hurt myself. This is the true beginning of great relationships, where we choose our actions by how it feels rather than how we "should" act.

As more of the inhabitants of this world enlighten, we will easily and spontaneously solve environmental, political, social, and economic crises from a whole new consciousness that sees possibilities we cannot now see. The current state of affairs is the natural product of the current collective consciousness and its consensus reality that limits what's possible. Once our thinking gets more up to speed with the Divine Intelligence within us, we more consistently operate at what is now thought of as genius level. Every person has the seeds of their own unique genius within.

We all have factions within our own selves that disagree or conflict with each other. It is that discord within each of us that manifests out there in the world as conflict and war. When we judge, loath, or criticize ourselves, and resist or reject aspects of ourselves instead of just experiencing them and allowing them to be, there is war within us. When we are disconnected from our Large Self that is always peaceful, there is war within. When there is struggle and unrest with our own families, it is the same energy as war.

Peace begins within each of us, with compassion and acceptance for ourselves—from a quiet, calm mind, allowing of all our parts and aspects. As all our scattered parts are accepted, valued, and experienced, they are soothed—they make peace. Then, from that peaceful and quiet place within ourselves, the love that is our true nature flows from us without trying. The heart flowers. From there it is a natural result to begin to authentically feel and give more love, appreciation, and compassion for our beloveds, families, co-workers, and friends. Then we begin to feel oneness with our city, our country, the world and so on, as this inner peace ripples out into the world. We are each a broadcast station for whatever energy we predominantly generate. Do not underestimate how powerful a generator you are.

Mother Teresa was asked for advice on how to promote world peace.
Her reply was, "Go home and love your family."

The logical extension of the inner peace we gain through Divine Openings is outer peace. Peace doesn't mean agreement. It can mean respectfully agreeing to disagree, even strongly.

Only from the Large Self can there be genuine relationship with a lover, a child, a parent or co-workers. Relationships from small-self-perspective are inauthentic and transactional, guarded, conflicted, conditional, needy, brittle, easily shattered, and lonely. From the Large Self, relationships are unconditional, allowing of differences, rich and deep, safe, rewarding, eternal and ever expanding. Unconditional love doesn't mean you stay with someone. Unconditional love means you allow someone to *be as they are and as they are not*. You love them no matter how it plays out in the physical. You love them from near or far as you choose.

Fully experience another's perspective, see the world through their eyes and feel the world through their perceptions—and you truly begin to relate. Nelson Mandela says it took him twenty-two years in prison to let go of his anger, see from the perspective of his "enemies," and make them his friends. Only then was he released, to transform his country and its people. He was not a perfect man; you don't have to be perfect to do great good.

Relating is different from relationship. "A relationship" is a thing to control or possess. "Relating" is a process that is allowing, flexible, alive, and active.

Call it a relationship and it is too easily perceived as something set in stone. Life is change, so if a relationship isn't changing, *it's not open and flowing*. Fear has us try to control it, preserve, or freeze it. Relate to your mother, your father, your lover in each moment, as an active process requiring your heart and your full presence. Decide to *experience* (not just conceptualize) true relating in relationship, and giving and receiving become barely distinguishable.

Compassion, love, and oneness cannot be successfully legislated or mandated. How successful have our laws and prisons been at mandating and controlling crime and terrorism? Trying to change people from the outside by controlling them is a short term fix at the very best. Fortunately, there is no need to force, manipulate, or legislate peace when it springs from within each individual authentically; as more and more individuals know their own Divinity and feel their oneness with everyone else, peace will spread. Enlightened beings naturally make choices and create solutions that reflect their knowing of who they truly are.

From there, getting along with, honoring and collaborating with other families, factions and eventually other countries is a natural flow rather than a figuring out of how-to's. There is no other way to act once we know who we are—when we've experienced our whole self, our Large Self.

Let go of the story of about what people are doing and be with your feeling response to it.
Once you can soften, accept, and allow everything, life is smooth and blissful no matter what is happening.

How Do I Clean Up My Relationships?

GRACE HELPS YOU and your Large Self guides you. Your intention and sincere willingness to get free are all you need. Divine Source is not going to force you to get free against your will. It is your choice, but you don't have to know *how* to do it, you just have to say, *I want it. Do it for me or show me how.* Then The Indweller provides the means and the how to's. Don't make it work. It's not complicated. Your job is just to relax, let go of resistance, and allow it to happen.

In a Houston workshop, in the silence in her own mind after her first Divine Opening, a participant saw, in her mind, a brief slide show featuring her deceased mother, who had not been kind to her. She felt the discord, felt it release, and "knew" it was done. Complete! She came to the workshop with the intention to move her life forward, but she didn't expect to resolve her relationship with her mother. Her Large Self knew how vital it is to clean up key relationships, and Divine Grace did the work. Many students had a similar "slide show" that provided instant resolution for them, devoid of the dramatic emotion of the original experiences. Some have just *felt something resolve* without knowing or seeing any details. Others hear and feel nothing during the Divine Opening, but then "something happens" in the coming days. One woman's dad called her for the first time in thirty years the day after a Divine Opening. She didn't feel "forgiveness." She felt love.

Some people need to read this book more than once to build up the willingness to clean up all relationships. I cannot tell you how much of a difference it makes. It changes your life.

God Doesn't Forgive!

A WOMAN PRAYED to God fervently for months for forgiveness for some awful things she had done. One night, exhausted from her suffering, she lay in bed and gave up, just hoping to die. Then she heard a voice saying, "I can never forgive you…" She panicked and began to wail. But the voice continued, "…because I never judged you."

The Presence doesn't judge you, punish you, or hold grudges. Humans do. I recently heard that an Amish mother whose child was killed in a school shooting declared that she would hold no grudges. To set an example that others could follow, she purchased thousands of erasers imprinted with the words "grudge eraser" and gave them away at media events.

People spontaneously open their hearts without effort to people they had shut out, sometimes after having a single Divine Opening. In the instant their perspective shifts to Large Self they wonder why it was so difficult or complicated to just let it go. Once that shift occurs, the word "forgiveness" doesn't begin to describe what happens. From that new consciousness, there is never anything to forgive, because your Large Self never judged in the first place.

After a Divine Opening, one woman was guided from within to list about ten people she'd been "trying to forgive" for years, and as she went down the list, one by one intending to "work on it"—she noticed there was nothing left to forgive! All that remained was peace and even love.

Think about it. Doesn't it sound a bit arrogant to say to someone, "I forgive you"? As if your small self ever held the right to judge them? And now you deign to say they're okay? I think of it now as "letting go" or "freeing myself." It's me choosing to return to Large Self perspective. I had been poking that old stick in my eye; now I put it down. I had been nursing that pain; now I walk on, a free woman.

It feels more accurate to me to say, "I've stopped judging you," than to say, "I forgive you."

Rather than, "I forgive you," try, "I give up judging you so I can be free."

Releasing Past Hurts

FIRST, SOFTEN around the painful feeling. Simply allow the feeling to be what it is, even if you don't like it. Stay focused on your body, breathing through the feeling, and ignore the story about it in my mind. Say to the other person in your own mind, "Letting go of hurts I've been clinging to *frees me* and stops the poisoning of my body and soul from resentment, anger, or sadness. I'm letting go of this *for me.*"

Sit quietly and speak inside your heart to anyone who has hurt you, living or dead. Tell them how you felt, and what you wanted from them. Don't go over the story. *Just say how you felt and what you wanted.* Period. "I felt worthless. I wanted to feel valued and loved."

One man went into the stillness inside and asked The Presence to be with him as he told his deceased father how hurt he had been when his father had beat him from childhood up to his teen years. He told his father that he had wanted to be hugged and praised. Love flooded him as he was freed from that burden, and for the first time he was shown how tortured his father had been.

Once you've done this, you will know if you need to say something to the real live person. And if you do speak to them, say it from the perspective of *how you felt and what you wanted*, rather than making it about them or what they did. Let go of their response—it doesn't matter—your freedom is guaranteed.

The only good use I've found for the word forgiveness is to forgive *myself*. Judging or condemning yourself is the most damaging thing you can do in all of creation.

You may forgive yourself now: "I forgive you for creating this. I love you."

Free Yourself, the Rest Will Follow

IF SOMEONE hurt you in the past, however painful it was, it is now history. You are learning how to attract something better in the future. Experience the emotion without the story, your vibration rises, you are free, and you don't attract that again. If you remain a victim and keep regenerating that emotion and vibration by telling and retelling the terrible story to yourself and others, *now who's hurting you?* You are hurting yourself over and over by continuing to hold onto that feeling. It's like poking a stick in your own eye to continue to dwell on that old hurt.

The chain of pain can end with you. You may stop carrying it now.

It's too difficult to try to figure out logically who hurt whom first, and why. The chain of pain passes down through thousands of generations—people who hurt you were themselves in pain of some kind, and so it goes, back into ancient history. But with ease and Grace it can end with you now. When you free yourself, it ripples out to humanity, even backwards and forwards in time.

You think you wanted others to be there for you, but what you really needed was to be there for yourself. Start being there for yourself right now, like a big brother or sister, even if no one else was there for you back then. This incredibly powerful decision changes your past, present, and future, and most importantly, it allows The Presence to be there fully for you.

In all situations, your first order of business is not to change them or
what they're doing—it's to be with your feeling response to it. Then everything opens up.

You are the only one you have any control over. Make the decision to let go, and let The Divine do the heavy lifting. Ask to know Truth, to know Oneness, to allow Life Source to flow fully through you. Ask for any obstacles to be moved. Working on it adds resistance to resistance so intend that this process occur for you with ease and grace. Experience, embrace, and breathe into that feeling without thinking about it, and let it rise and resolve.

It's *your love* that's been shut off, and when you let it flow again, you are liberated, restored to your true Self. Do it for you, not for the other person. If your love pipeline stays closed, your life energy is pinched off, you contract, and you are out of alignment with your Large Self. Your Large Self never has to forgive, because your Large Self never judges. The only person it makes any sense to forgive is you. To remove the negative charge, say, "I forgive myself for creating that reality."

Relationships are an important part of what life in this dimension is about, and they are one of the keys to your freedom. By letting go of hurts, you are *not* saying it was OK—you are saying that you choose being happy over being right. You are claiming your power to free yourself. As you practice being *there for yourself*, you find your Large Self was already there, waiting for you, calling you to freedom. As you get back in alignment with your Large Self, everything looks and feels different.

Even if no one was ever there for you, now YOU may be there for you.

With compassion (not judgment) I tell you these next two stories, to make the point that even with the blissful free rides Grace gives, we must sustain our enlightenment and bring it down to earth. The *conscious mind piece* of Divine Openings is only about 10% of the total, but it is necessary for our awakening. Remember the friend I mentioned who, before we met, had a very flashy cosmic oneness experience you might think would be anyone's ultimate, end-all bonanza? She was in orgasmic ecstasy for months, but it may surprise you that once it was over, her life didn't change much. She did get contented living simply on little money, but she still holds family grudges, justifies it, doesn't accept that she creates her reality, is accident-prone (matching the belief that problems in her life are accidental), and although she is gorgeous and sexy, lovers don't stay. She still reads literally hundreds of spiritual books, but still isn't willing to feel lower vibrations and claim authorship of her life. "Energy junkies" chase the cosmic energy highs, but try to avoid ordinary feelings, denying they create them, or blaming them on others.

A PhD psychologist who didn't read this book had a spontaneous cosmic explosion of ecstasy and oneness that lasted weeks, long before we met. Afterward, he went back to resenting ex-spouses, continued attracting heartbreaks, and teaches Law Of Attraction but struggles with living it. The awakening is permanent only when we do our part to bring it "down to earth" by practicing the conscious mind piece. This book and our multi-media online courses guide you.

Grace tosses you aloft like a dove into flight.
Your conscious choices keep you there.

This activity, along with the Divine Opening that follows, frees you and restores your flow. Your job is simply to get out of the way and allow it to happen—to be willing. *There's no work to do.* If you notice Divine Openings becoming work you have slipped back into the old toil and struggle paradigm and progress will be difficult.

In your notebook, make a list of people in your life, past and present, living and dead, where your love is even a little bit withheld, or not fully flowing.

> **The key relationships are parents, siblings, children, family members, spouses, ex-spouses, and business associates, living or dead.**
> Next are business associates and friends.
> Include yourself—is love fully flowing for yourself? Do you adore yourself as The Divine does?
> How about government leaders, your president, politicians?

Enemies of your nation? Terrorists? People who pollute the environment?

People at work? Rich, greedy people? Poor, lazy people?

People who are closed-minded, mean, perverted?

People who put other people down?

Those who let you down, broke your heart, or you broke theirs.

People who clearly did you wrong.

Ones where you're on the good guys' side and they're clearly (really!) the bad guys.

Anyone who hooks you, or that you have an emotional charge on.

If your list is blank and your love flows freely to everyone on the planet, first check if you're being honest! If it's true, sit and enjoy this unconditional love radiating from you. Your intention might be, "How do I go deeper?" or, "Make me a beacon."

Remember: all the people on your list have been in the grip of Ancient Mind, just as you were, and their thoughts and "choices" were often not their own. Remember they too wanted to feel and act better, and be free of the bondage to their mind and emotions. But they could not, just as you could not always do it. Ask your Large Self for help in raising your vibration about relationships so that you may be liberated and your enlightenment can fully flower. You don't have to do the work, just be willing to turn it over to The Indweller, and it's all taken care of.

APPLY IT NOW: Stop reading and do this now. Reading doesn't make it happen, feeling it through and experiencing it in the circumstances of your life does:

Place your hand over your heart and breathe through your heart.

Let it be the hand of your Large Self, The Indweller, The Divine Presence.

Soften around the feelings and allow them to be whatever they are, without trying to fix them or make them go away. Dive In.

Allow any hurt, disappointment, or loss to comes to mind with a key person in your life or past.

Express very softly, in a whisper, *what feeling you wanted that you didn't get.*

Receive the next Divine Opening on the coming page.

(On a separate occasion do this for all those *you have been small with.*)

Note in your journal over the next few weeks what you notice about your relationships. You may have felt nothing extraordinary in the activity and Divine Opening, yet relationships open up by themselves, love flows, or you just feel okay about it now. Celebrate any movement and you'll get more.

Large Self Perspective

FROM YOUR LARGE SELF perspective you recognize that you create your reality. Don't "blame yourself" in a small-self, victim-like way. Be soft and kind to yourself. Take your power back first, and get your vibration up before you take too much responsibility. Moving any lower emotions as you feel them helps you authentically rise up out of them.

From Large Self, declare, "I created that," and feel your power swell. You don't need to know why you created it. The answer will come if you need to know.

Don't analyze, push yourself, or struggle with this. It may be that upon the third or fourth reading of the book, this will suddenly seem natural and effortless. You can celebrate that day when it comes!

There is no hurry. Your Large Self patiently calls to you, yet judges you not.

When you own that you created it, you get your power back.

This book helps you pass through Portal 1, out of suffering, to create momentum toward your peace, stability, and happiness. It's to get your Large Self in the driver's seat more of the time. Divine Openings is not supposed to be about speed bumps and hairballs forever—that's old paradigm stuff. You can be absolutely sure Grace is doing its 90%, but you must use your Free Will to do your 10%. Your 10% is mostly softening, letting go, and using the conscious mind material—it's not hard work.

~ Are you still listening to your mind'?

~ Are you actually doing the activities?

~ You're not processing and working on yourself anymore, right?

A couple of times I've used tough love, my in-your-face cowgirl guru mode and said to a student, "*Make a decision!* Get mad if you need to! *Decide* to stop letting your mind run your life. *Decide now* to keep the nose tipped up, and decide that *nothing*—is worth tipping the nose of your plane down for long! This is your precious life. *Only you* can make this choice. You have Free Will." They got the wake-up call, made their choice, and moved to a whole new level. Make choices that nourish and support you in every way in every part of your life.

For accelerated progress or more support, the online courses are always there for you if you choose. The resonance field is amplified when you hear my voice vibrations in the audios and videos I've recorded while teaching and counseling. The first course includes my reading of this entire book as an Audio Book. Voluminous material I've created (and continue to create) since this book was written helps keeps you engaged and focused as the world tries its best to distract you. As I'm channeling those teachings, the Energy alone is palpable, but what comes through me in answer to students' specific needs and desires on every topic will speak to you as if meant for you.

You may enjoy life *right now.*

Witnessing My Smaller Self

I DON'T RECOMMEND that you go looking for negativity in yourself, or anyone, *ever, at any time.* But you'll feel when you're vibrating lower because Divine Openings makes it increasingly *intolerable* to stay in lower vibrations. It will feel awful, and it should! Don't make it bad or wrong, don't be afraid of it or resist it. The vibration will rise with your loving, gentle Large Self embrace. There is nothing to do. The "bad" feeling plus the desire to feel better propels you toward what you want.

The darkness is not your true self. It's only what you experience when your smaller, denser self closes its eyes to the light. Turn on the light! Witness and softly accept the small self, be with it, and soon, although you remain human and imperfect, you are not run by it anymore.

Our positive spiritual personas and pretensions are just as insidious as any negative personas. As I asked The Presence for relief from some false selves I had built up, I didn't like what I felt and saw, but was willing to be with it. Then as I naturally pivoted from what I didn't want to what I did want, a wave of strong desire to be more authentic washed over me. How had I not seen how false it was to pretend to be more cheerful than I really was? How had I not seen the degree of my alienation from other people? A transactional mentality showed itself. There was loss-prevention strategy in some of my decisions that made no sense in my rich and blessed life. I was kind to myself and didn't condemn, so those layers of masks fell off, leaving me tremendously relieved and renewed. In the light of consciousness, the vibration rose, without any work.

Once awakening begins, we are glad to see these things! My job was to relax and receive—and let the Divine do the heavy lifting. Lately, all I have to do is focus lightly on something I want, and it develops fairly quickly. There is no more working on myself. I'm on "automatic evolution," and you are too; as soon as you stop seeking and let it be this easy, the desire is often granted overnight. Appreciation poured out of me for yet another degree of freedom and authenticity. I'm still not perfect, but it's not about perfection, it's about the ever-unfolding, evolving journey.

There's no need to figure out or fix your human imperfection.
Fall in love with your perfect imperfection.

As Awakening Unfolds

THE BEST NEWS is: as you become more expanded, you will have less and less difficulty keeping your altitude up. The only reason we ever had any difficulty with heavy feelings is that we'd resisted feeling them fully and had a huge backlog of density. We'd been taught some feelings were bad, or we thought we couldn't bear to feel them. We'd inhibited them or stopped the flow altogether. We did anything to avoid painful feelings. I know, sometimes it hurt so much, and they seemed to go on forever! Well, no more.

Feelings can now flow through you as they were designed to do, quickly, easily, without analysis, story, or processing. Live and feel fully. Allow everything to move through you. You'll still have the full range of emotions. There is still contrast. You still like some things more than others. You just don't get as hooked or suffer over it. This is equanimity.

You still get angry, sad, disappointed, and frustrated from time to time, and as you fully experience each emotion, it relaxes upward again. The more time you spend at higher vibrations, the more Law of Attraction holds you up there, and the more "rubberized" you get. You snap back up into the higher vibrations fast—as if a rubber band connects you to the top of the Instrument Panel. The longer you vibrate up there, the stronger and thicker that rubber band gets. Even deep negative emotion can give way to bliss very quickly when it's embraced.

Five minutes of meditation now goes deeper than an hour used to. A quick moment to dip within and shift to Large Self perspective can bring quiet bliss, or set off peals of laughter.

Enlightenment is different from saintliness where you never get angry and you always have your halo on. The Dali Lama is known never to suffer fools or time-wasters; he'll walk out of the room, terminating the interview abruptly. I know one enlightened man who smokes cigars and drinks whiskey at times. You could even be a blunt, grouchy enlightened character who tells off-color jokes and annoys people. Your uniqueness remains or even increases; oneness does not mean sameness or uniformity. Different perspectives are valued. Enlightenment does not mean perfection. Please drop your old stereotypes and be *you*. This is a whole new world.

We come here for the full range of individual expressions this dimension offers.

The Evolution of Who You Are

SIX MONTHS AFTER creating a more personal concept of God, I evolved into a state where I didn't feel God as separate from myself at all. It expanded from a mere concept to a real experience. I know I'm not *all* of what God is, but I'm part of God and one with God. So now my daily dialogue with The Presence feels for all practical purposes like talking with myself—my Larger Self. That's now normal. What stands out as odd now is the voice and feelings of my small self.

This can be disconcerting at first if you've spent a lifetime looking to "outside" authorities: parents, experts, leaders, doctors, and a God who is "out there," above and separate from you calling all the shots. If you're accustomed to being told what is right and wrong, what is good and bad, and what is the "best" course of action to take, it's like taking your training wheels off and riding the bike alone. But that fear is just the remnants of small-self perception. We are never alone or separate!

Becoming your own inner-guided authority is a spiritually mature stance to take. What if this life (and The Creator itself) is more experimental, unfinished, and adventurous than we believed, and welcomes your help creating the future, giving you carte blanche to do whatever you like, and eternity to try different things? That might make some people nervous, especially if they require rules and absolute black and white answers to everything, but for those of you on the leading edge, it's exhilarating.

The good news about Self Realization is that you are responsible for your entire reality.
The bad news about Self Realization is that you are responsible for your entire reality.

I'm joking. There is no bad news. When we let go to the Large Self, there is no burdensome responsibility to micro-manage or strategize our reality. We are carried by a Flow of Life that easily relieves us of much of the work and struggle. Once we take that first step to open our eyes and claim our power, and let go of the details, the rest is easy. Divine Intelligence orchestrates our lives. We still co-create it with our Free Will, and we still take action, but the more we let go of tension and resistance, the easier it goes. We still pick up the hammer and hit the nail, but our aim is true, we hit our own thumb less often, and life is fun.

It is true that when the small self gets hold of the concept that *it* is God, trouble ensues. But that is one of the risks of this game, and you can handle it. And if you crash and burn, no worries—get up and have another go at it. We are all far too serious about this game called Life.

How would you live if you were sure you couldn't lose?

Divine Opening

CONTEMPLATE the photographic work of art for two minutes,
and then close your eyes and experience.

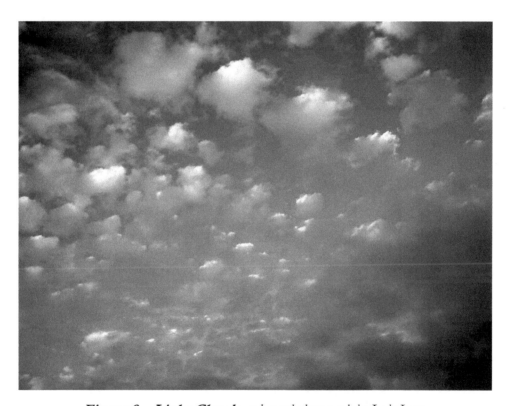

*Figure 8—**Light Clouds**, enhanced photograph by Lola Jones.*

A New Way to "Work"

IN THE ALL-TOO-SHORT story of the Garden of Eden, there was a time when Man lived in ease. Food grew on trees, life was easy, and there was no work. Whether you believe that particular story is literal or a metaphor, most people agree on one point: somewhere along the way, man went astray. And ever since then, through countless generations, many daily lives have been long chapters of struggle, toil, and conflict.

Take a moment to review the "plot" of all the movies you can think of, and you will find that almost all revolve around a problem or a long struggle, and after much difficulty our hero/heroine prevails over the challenges. Very short scene of happy hero. End of movie. Two hours of pain and struggle, fighting, or conflict in great detail, with a short nod at the end to the "happily ever after," which we never actually get to see play out in detail, so we don't have much evidence that it exists. The respite is short in any case, and is followed by another sequel that resumes with more struggle and strife. Hero prevails, fade to black. And that's entertainment! Think about it! That's our conditioned unconscious expectation, and no one questions that we call that entertainment!

We're not conscious of how deeply we believe life is that way—a long struggle, with very short bouts of happiness. Some movies don't even give us the happy ending (those are considered the more "realistic" or "important" movies.) The Academy Awards favors those and snubs the happy, funny, "frivolous" movies. We believe in suffering and happiness is suspect. We don't notice these assumptions—we just live them. We don't have nearly as many role models for "happy most of the time" as we do for "strugglers and overcomers of hardship." The fascinating real life story of the racehorse Seabiscuit, the book, and the movie are all about overcoming crushing obstacles, with a little triumph and happiness sprinkled in here and there. And that's what we used to call "real life."

It's all right there in Technicolor in our movies. Rather than dwell further on how life lost its ease, let's skip right to the happy ending, which this time will not be short. The ancient story can change for you if you choose to shake off the mass hallucinations and create your own story.

The future you experience hinges upon the choices you make today. Reality is multi-dimensional, and every single person on this planet *experiences a different version of reality*. You really do live in a different reality than your parents, co-workers, or friends. We all have infinite potential, but some of us allow ourselves more possibilities, while others, to fit in and be comfortable, cling to the illusions and prescribed limits of consensus reality.

As you play with this more and more you'll notice that people act differently in the new realities you create. You and others look different in the new reality. Things work differently in the new reality. When people talk of doom and gloom—or this or that eminent global disaster—I'll say, "That's not *my* reality." I can't change everyone else's reality, but I can sure show them how.

For those who choose to claim their inner power, there will be an unlimited choice of realities. In the coming times work will consist of each of us doing what we were born to do, and enjoying it. Whether you are a truck driver, a hairstylist, a ditch digger, or a doctor, work will be an out-flowing of your genius and passion, an exercise in self-expression, a way to flow life force in a way you enjoy. You will play in this material reality, not to survive, but to create, experiment, savor, expand, and master your chosen endeavor. You will not spend your life making a living, which is survival, but making a life, which is creativity.

This return to The Garden is not an end goal. It is just another phase of evolution. We've entered a fast-moving new dimension of evolution that is unprecedented in recorded history.

The wooden plow is primitive compared to the giant combines of today. Today's fantastic reality was inconceivable to the medieval king. Similarly, we have no way of imagining from here what is coming. But it's fun to try—it stretches your sense of possibility and imagination! We will one day co-create even more fully with the Essence Of Life, not only on this Earth, but to create entirely new worlds in new dimensions. How would you like to be a "world designer"? You learn more about this in Level Two (it's all about joy and creating for the fun of it), and by Jumping The Matrix, which is essentially Level Four, you'll be playing with alternate realities outside of time and space. Most of the new developments go into those Online Retreat Courses because I enjoy multi-media—audios, videos, colorful graphics, and art are so much fun. The web is "alive," flexible, and perfect for the way I create, improve, add to, and update things continuously.

Do what you love, and love what you do. It feels good flowing through you.

Life Proves Our Beliefs

WHEN A FRIEND lamented some manifestations he wasn't enjoying, he realized how his guardedness and defensiveness was bringing more manifestations that validated his belief in struggle, conflict and the need for guardedness. Life always brings us proof of what we believe is true. Then people say, "I can't just *pretend* it isn't true because it's real. See, it happened *again! Proof that it's real!*"

But a truth is only true because you believed it and collected big box of evidence for it, or a whole society believed it and you bought it. Then Law of Attraction made it truer.

It was understandable that his background as a martial artist had ingrained in him the need to be constantly wary of attack, and we talked about how that vibration had attracted so much discord with other people—lovers, business partners, friends. He saw it, but wasn't at all sure what to do. While it's usually easy for me to stay in cool, calm, Large Self perspective with students, I felt an emotional charge talking with my friend that day.

Soon it became clear why, and I received a gift of awareness too. Later that day, wells of tears began to flow out of me with the sudden recognition that I was somewhat defended too, but it just manifested differently with me; it was more hidden, and I didn't let the conflicts and guardedness show. I had played it out less overtly, and it was less damaging in my life, but there it was nevertheless. In facilitating clarity for him, I saw myself more clearly. I breathed easier on that soft, clear night as I let down the walls. I watched him become a little more open and less guarded with the world. His businesses thrived. My own romantic relationship deepened. A friend who had harshly criticized me months before called and renewed our estranged friendship. Life opens more doors when our hearts soften.

Whatever you believe (and so vibrate) will repeatedly prove itself to you.

Boxes of Beliefs: What is "True"?

YOU THINK LIFE CREATES YOUR BELIEFS, but actually your beliefs create your life. You think circumstances create your emotions, but that is backwards too— your vibration creates your circumstances, and after a string of similar events are magnetized to you, you develop a belief and encounter more similar circumstances.

Our minds love to organize our experience and make rules about what's true so we feel in control. We develop beliefs by attracting similar things and feelings over and over. We vibrationally attract "proof" of those beliefs, which we file away in the boxes in our minds. The boxes then attract more evidence that "prove" our beliefs. Any box of evidence you've collected is constantly attracting more evidence to prove it is true, even if the belief is not true. Proofs keep accumulating.

There are big problems with this. We oversimplify things and distort them to make them fit into "boxes" in our minds. We believe the "proofs." We use our boxes of past experiences to know what is true and real rather than in the moment guidance from our Large Selves.

If you believe your sister is lazy, you will collect evidence of it, and delete counter-evidence because it doesn't fit in your neat little box. If you believe people can't be trusted, that belief actively attracts people who can't be trusted. I don't have that belief or box of evidence, so I rarely attract people who can't be trusted. I am trusting, but still *discerning*. I accidentally left a purse with eight-hundred dollars cash in it in a disco in Mexico and got it back the next day. I've dropped fifty dollars on the floor of a store and had it turned in. I've taken rides from strangers. I constantly prove my box of evidence that I'm safe, and all I do is use my intuition wisely to avoid trouble. That box works. No problem. What about boxes of evidence that limit you, hold you back, or inhibit success and relationships?

I used to have boxes of proof that I wasn't lovable. The experiences I used to have in relationships when I lived from that box now seem alien to me, although they were reality at one time. Now I feel completely lovable and secure, and am well loved; that's simply not an issue.

Everything is true—for someone, but it doesn't have to be true for you. I live in another reality now, outside that box. You wouldn't read a 1950s book about medicine or rocket science. The truths in your more expanded reality are "truer" than your old, more limiting truths.

Another example of this is a man with boxes full of evidence that his father was bad, and that soon extended to "males in authority are bad." The evidence may be factual and "true," but that box just attracts more abusive authorities. Such beliefs can ruin our lives without our understanding what is happening.

Some people have boxes of evidence that they are shy, or can't make money, or aren't attractive. Some have beliefs, supported by boxes of evidence, that they don't get guidance, or they are not smart, that the world is doomed, or that work is hard. I overheard a man in a coffee shop say, "That stuff about doing what you love and the money will follow—I tried it, and it's not true." I thought, "How sad. It's always been true for me. But he's right for himself because his boxes are full of proof and getting bigger."

Once you bust the box, you can just let go to the flow. The new paradigm has us receive the guidance or information we need in the moment that it is needed. You don't need boxes, just as you don't need prior experience of a route to take a trip. Just tune into your Instrument Panel and follow your guidance moment by moment. The mind wants boxes of proof and evidence for security but now you know that's fear-based. You don't even need "faith" with your Large Self to guide you.

Live in the now, not from boxes.

Please relax around all this if you have any boxes that feel too big to bust by yourself. Just ask your Large Self to do it, soften around the belief, and let it happen. Grace makes all things possible—even things we have struggled with for years.

APPLY IT NOW: How many boxes of "true evidence" do you have that aren't helping you? In your notebook, write some things you believe that limit you, and ask for Divine help in letting go of that evidence. You could also Dive In or prostrate for a little boost.

How Do You Know What Is Possible?

HOW DO YOU know if something is "possible" or "impossible" for you? Do you refer to the Internet, books, science, statistics, and your boxes? That's how most people decide if something is possible or impossible for them or anyone. Cancer? AIDS? Oh, that's incurable. Blindness? Incurable. Be prosperous? No way. Living simply? Not possible for me. Everyone on the planet being fed? Nope, there is only so much to go around.

If you have never experienced it before, or have never seen anyone on the planet do it, all the data in your boxes might say, "No, you can't do that, it is impossible," when Divine guidance might say, "Go for it, you can do it." How can we evolve above and beyond what's ever been done if we must have boxes of evidence that something is possible first? This reinforces how important it is to give more credence to our own visions than to outer evidence boxes and past experience.

The earth is round, man can fly, the four-minute mile, talk to people halfway around the world—all these were once impossible, and that was backed up by the best science of the day. Now they're not only possible, they're *mundane.* For much more on boxes, beliefs, and freedom from them, search www.DivineOpenings.com for the article, "Reality: Some Dis-Assembly Required."

Give over to your Large Self anything that is too big for your small self.

Give Your To-Do List to God

I STILL MAKE to-do lists and vision boards, but it's very different now. I think of it as putting it on the "God list" as one client dubbed it. Then I only do what I feel moved, inspired, and pulled to do, or must do for a deadline, like pay bills. Once it's on the "God list" it's done in the Non-Physical. Then I put it away and forget it! Instead of making myself do the items on my list, I stay tuned for inspired thoughts or urges to act, which for me are abundant. I love accomplishing things. If I think something needs action, I feel the vibration and check if it feels "ripe" or "cooked." I don't do much until I feel the tailwind behind it or even pushing it. If it feels sluggish it's not time yet, and no amount of action will make it successful. If the energy isn't cooked yet, action is wasted. When my energy is aligned with my Large Self on that subject, it's time to act.

I love it for big projects, big challenges, finding someone to do things I don't do well, creating money, finding just the right item, and receiving solutions to things I have no idea how to handle. I put all the mundane things as well as the "too big for me to handle" things on the mental God list. If I'm feeling resistant, I put it on *paper*. It is very efficient. A lot of the heavy lifting gets done by the universe, by someone else, or it ends up not really needing to be done at all. Something often comes along that works better with less effort than you thought.

Let The Divine do the heavy lifting.

APPLY IT NOW:

1. Make a list of all the people with whom you think it is impossible to resolve issues. Then let go.

2. Write a list of heart's desires "too big" or complicated for you to accomplish, then let go.

Anything is possible for your Large Self. Just give it over and "be willing."

Where Does Action Come In?

YOU'RE TUNING IN MORE FINELY to your inner guidance and becoming less dependent on outside answers—but it's still a physical world. Don't just sit at your desk and expect everything to come to you from within, or for free, although it might. Yes, some action is required to create in this physical dimension. We came here to manipulate matter, communicate with other people, and mold the physical clay with our hands, and we enjoy that. If we'd wanted just to create in the Non-Physical realms, where everything appears instantly with just a thought, we'd have stayed in the Non-Physical.

On Earth, part of the game is material manifestation. We have more fun and less fatigue when we take advantage of the fact that 99.9% of creation is done with energy, vibration, focus, and intention, and only that last fraction is physical manifestation. I've spent all this time with you on the energy part. Now that your energy is up, and you're allowing the Flow of Life to carry you along, you'll feel inspired to act. Begin by taking one step. You may only be led one step at a time and there may be many forks in the road.

If action is hard, are you following your guidance or your mind? People say writing is hard, yet because I write from guidance, I find it exhilarating, effortless, and flowing. I relish writing and often can't stop. My Large Self does the writing and I let go and let it work through me. I get reminded and inspired reading my own work, and listening to my own audios, and because it comes from my Large Self, not the small me. You can let The Divine do the heavy lifting in any profession.

You've said what you want. Now your Large Self offers you guidance and leads you to what you need to do. You're nudged in the direction of people who have the skills and information you don't have—the great babysitter, the best accountant, the supplies you need, the best vacation deal, or the person who builds you a website that does a lot of the work for you.

One of those found me! Lee took a live Divine Openings Level One with his wife Brooke early on in Divine Openings. I didn't know he did websites, and he didn't know I was looking for a new one. A month later, he emailed me with a proposed plan for the exact website that I'd been shopping for. He proposed we trade the Five-Day Silent Retreat for himself and his wife. We started that week. Within two months I had a sophisticated new website, and within four months it was doing 90% of my work for me. Things started going *even better* in my absence through the worldwide web!

Life brings you opportunities to co-create with others to accomplish goals, have fun, exercise, build a company, or tune up your car. It prompts you in the perfect timing to clean up a relationship, say hello to a stranger, make the phone call, hire the person, read the article, and follow the trail. The most natural next step always shows up once the energy is lined up. Are you open to see it?

Your job is to tune in, feel the timing, and then take the guided physical action. I feel what I call a "smoothness" when it's time to act. It feels good in my body. The doubts aren't there.

My book that follows this one, *Watch Where You Point That Thing: Mastering Your Power of Intention*, continues where this book leaves off and further develops your ability to create and manifest with pure intention.

Guidance is always being offered. Are you tuned in?

Follow Your Guidance

ONE CLIENT, who ended up being initiated as a Divine Openings Guide, had huge awakenings after her first session. A hairball or two were coughed up. In the first week, awful recurring scenarios popped into her head where people she didn't know were abusing her or trying to control her. In her long-practiced habit of "spiritual bypassing" instead of feeling, she tried to "wrap them in white light and make them go away." They kept coming back.

As we talked about it, I intuited that she had not been allowed to express anger as a child. For all her life, when someone made her feel powerless, she could not let herself use anger to blast up the Altimeter. She had been trying in vain all her life to do the spiritual bypass on her negative feelings. "Just think love and light." Well, that's too big a jump from powerless to love, and most people can't make it stick. They fall back down, and then feel they failed.

I had her be with the feelings, starting from powerlessness, then move on up through anger. I coached her to face the abusers in her own mind, get angry, and tell them they could *not* abuse and control her anymore! Relief quickly followed.

Then I guided her to feel the feelings to the core, but drop the characters and the story. They had served their purpose. I led her deeper into the Diving In process. The feelings rose in vibration, and the "abusers" stopped appearing. Then she was authentically up in love, light and power, and could stay there.

Spiritual people sometimes, wanting to "be good," don't want to *ever* have, admit, or feel the lower vibrations, thinking that's failure. I see highly advanced spiritual people stay stuck until they learn to embrace, allow, and flow their emotions. Once you embrace them, you rise out of them.

The main point of my sharing this story, though, is that those visions were that woman's Divine guidance! We're looking for angels and listening for the booming voice of God, but from powerlessness, what God often sends you is the impetus to get angry to get your power back. Once she knew that, she not only felt great—she trusted that negative feelings do have a purpose. She began to honor and move them, not try to make them go away.

At the third session, I knew the next level was about to pop. She was so revved up, she was running ninety miles an hour. Usually over-revved people are running from something, and it's usually feelings. My sense was that she had been running ahead of her body all her life. And who can blame her? Who would want to be with a bad feeling they don't know how to handle? But now you have help from Grace. I soothed her, and she was ready to share that there was abuse in her childhood. She had been learning to Dive In and be with it, but this subject was still daunting. So I guided her through simply feeling it, not analyzing it or telling the story, and the old, dreaded emotion was soon, as she described it, a pile of ashes. Once again, she was ecstatic. She'll be able to dive in on her own now.

Guidance doesn't usually occur as the voice of a spirit guide or God—it doesn't always sound like you might expect it to. It might begin as a lower emotion that ultimately leads you upwards on the Instrument Panel to inspiration and action. When you're high on the Instrument Panel guidance often feels like pure bliss that merrily calls you down a certain trail. In any case, follow it!

Guidance will look and sound different depending on where you are on Instrument Panel.

Inspired Action

INSPIRED ACTION IS efficient and it feels more like it's carrying you. One hour of inspired action replaces thousands of hours of busyness, or I-should-do-this, or hard work. Now of course if you're building a stone fireplace, you must pick up stones and put the mortar between them. But if it's inspired action you'll thrill to the physical movement, the newly forming creation, and the sore muscles. You came here to build with stones and mortar, juggle numbers, take care of business, and wash dishes, not to float in the ethers. Enjoy delicious action. And when the feeling changes, take a break.

How do you know when an action that comes to mind is inspired? When the mind is quiet and peaceful most of the time, just about anything that comes in and feels good is inspired thought. Remember, the voice of The Divine sounds just like yours, only smarter. Most of my thoughts are inspired, guided, nurturing, or uplifting now. Sometimes my mind is not that active. When thoughts do run to the negative, I turn away from them, toward the direction I want to go. At a certain point, you may hear almost nothing inside—that's good—that means you're out of the way and Grace can easily lead you, so just move with the flow.

I compare my old mind to a cluttered airport runway with trash all over it. Your Large Self is always dropping gift packages on the runway, sending guidance. But when the runway is cluttered with junk we can't find the valuable packages in all the garbage. In the past I would muck around in the mind-garbage on the runway, not being able to decide what was valuable, and would get confused.

Being creative, I often have so many ideas I can't do them all. I can scatter my efforts too much, do too much action for too little result, or give up in overwhelm. All that action kept me tired.

Once Divine Openings cleared the clutter off the runway, it was different. When a Divine inspiration came in for a landing, it was easy to spot it out there all alone, and there was no doubt whatsoever if it was an "important" idea or action. Now I know exactly which ones are the inspired ideas, and which ones merit my priority attention. They stand out like neon signs on that clear funway… runway. (Interesting typo—I decided to leave it in there.)

Even when my mind is busy, if my altitude is high and if it's high quality I listen to it. A busy mind can be very productive, but you still need silent rests. If you get too many ideas all at once, write them down to capture them, then put them away. The timing will come to do them, or the universe will do much of it for you, *or you'll get the feeling you wanted without doing anything.*

If the guidance is not clear and I'm not inspired, I don't act unless it's absolutely essential. I wait until all the pieces show up, and they do. I pay the bills and taxes on time whether I'm inspired or not, of course, but in matters where I have choice of timing, if there is confusion, resistance, or I'm not feeling good about it, I don't act or make decisions until there is clarity and inspiration. Uninspired action from the small self, without alignment with Large Self, is often futile, wasted action. Money, time, and energy thrown at a project out of fear or need are wasted.

If you're low on the Instrument Panel when you think about a task, that's a message: "Raise altitude before taking action!" Motivational speakers tell us to take massive action. We already work longer hours than we have at any time in recent history, thinking that more action equals more results and more money. A quick look at the richest and poorest people in the world will tell you more work doesn't necessarily equal more money. Then again, when your action is inspired and you love the work, action is magically effective!

When you create your life in the easier "go with the tailwind" way, people who are out there working themselves to death may call you lazy, but you simply cannot please everyone. Let them do it their way and do what feels right for you. The old Puritan work ethic says punishing work and suffering are virtuous. The "joy ethic" says work because it feels good, produce because it's satisfying, act when you're in alignment with your Large Self, and get to the party that's already laid out for you!

Procrastination or sluggishness is often your Large Self telling you that your energy is not yet lined up to your Large Self's level on the subject at hand, so why waste the action? When your resistance on that subject has relaxed and your altitude on it is high, you will suddenly feel energized and compelled to action. This is letting go and letting God. Not everything has to be done this instant. That's your small self's judgment, some parental voice, or some goal-setting book you've read. Work, even hard work, is exhilarating when you're in the flow.

If you're not in control of the timing because you work for someone else, or there's an emergency or deadline, do your best to align energy before acting, and things will still go smoothly.

So, act, yes. But get your altitude up and point the nose where you want to go first. Otherwise you're flying into a headwind. You can't buck the natural forces of the universe—it just makes you tired. Are you doing what your heart desires or are you following someone else's idea of "success"?

Action and sweat can be fulfilling and rewarding. If it's not, look at where you might be out of alignment with your Large Self. The same action that feels heavy right now may feel light once you've raised your altitude. Change your attitude toward it. Find some joy in it (EN-joy it.) Imagine yourself at the party—things look and feel different from there. It's a different dimension, literally.

In the midst of action, if you begin to slide down the Altimeter or grind your gears—STOP. Relax, take a break, breathe, release resistance, and re-align your energy. Tip the nose up and point it where you want to go. Stop looking at the obstacles. Reset your course toward your desire.

Give the big tasks over to God, let go, and wait for guidance. Go do something that feels good, and you'll return to the task refreshed. Forgetting it for a while releases resistance.

Energy, intention, and alignment pave the way. Action follows that smoothed path.

The "It's Not Here Yet" Syndrome

YOU WOULD RECEIVE everything you want—and enjoy the ride there—if you would just relax, let go of the past, and let the flow take you. All that you want would come in time. Each time you say, "It's not here yet," it is delayed, because you have vibrated in opposition to what you want. You have sent the delivery truck back to the warehouse.

Whether it's deeper enlightenment, more love, a wonderful home, or a dream job, the best way to let it come more quickly is by appreciating any part of it that you already have. If you want a lover, think of all the other types of love you already have, or remember the best parts of past loves, and appreciate it deeply. Then Life can match you up with more of it. If you can't find any love in your past to feel, there's a clue. All your active vibrations are dominated by the "bad" feelings about your exes and your past. That's why you don't have love now. Maybe other things are more important to you, and you're splitting your intentions and don't realize it. You may value your freedom and you believe love will curtail it. If you want your freedom very powerfully, freedom wins out over love.

Be with the fact that you don't like the situation as it is, but lighten your grip on it. Gripping and control is resistance to the flow that would bring it to you! You can want something too "badly." If you spent all day daydreaming pleasantly about only the having of it, it would come. But if you're feeling "bad" about not having it, you are creating not having it. The more you feel the *lack* of it, the longer it is in coming. If you radiate lack energy Life matches it with more lack. If you can't want it in a "good" way, just don't think about it at all. Do something else. Removing attention releases resistance.

If you're working too hard on anything, take a break from it and do not think about it. If you want a great job, focus every day on the best parts of your current job. Appreciate your current job. "I do love working with Joan." "The hours are nice." In the financial world "appreciation" means your money has compounded. It means the same thing in the vibrational world.

Appreciation compounds your vibrational assets.

Savor the waiting for it. Start saying *(and feeling)*, "I feel it coming." "It's almost here." "Won't it be nice when it's here? What will it be like?"

Don't take score too soon. Only take score when the score is in your favor. If it's not in your favor, delay taking score. Skew the score. Find evidence that it's coming, and delete evidence that it isn't. Most of the quality of your day-to-day life will depend on what you focus on. So next time you find yourself observing that it isn't here yet, pivot to what you do have, and feel appreciation for it.

Daydream about the new job. It doesn't matter whether you try on new jobs in your imagination, or remember past good jobs, you will create it faster if you *feel like you already have it*. Lack attracts lack. Abundance attracts abundance. That's why the rich get richer and the poor get poorer.

Look for every opportunity to create love, humor, fun, and adventure. Radiate that, take steps toward it, and then let it in! That will work out a whole lot better than complaining it isn't here.

Keep making peace with where you are now, and now, and now. Say to yourself things like, "I am where I am! Where else could I be? Today is the product of yesterday's vibration and altitude. Tomorrow is the product of today's choices feelings, intentions, actions, dreams and visions."

You are where you are, and wherever you are is okay, because now you know how to get anywhere you want to go! Feel the instant relief in that?

Enlightenment is remembering your true essence that you're playing hide and seek from. As you open up to receive more Grace, you recover more of your essence and power. Your job is to relax and stay out of the way.

Each time you get impatient with a plateau, or bored with your old successes, stop and appreciate how far you've come. There will always be more you want as long as you're alive.

Being mad at yourself is far more damaging than being mad at someone else. Your Large Self is never mad at you, so if you are, you are not aligned with your Large Self. The Presence sees you as perfect, although evolving, right now. Agree with that! If you must get mad, get mad at something or someone, or even God (who can take it.) Anger gives you energy to move up the Instrument Panel. The moment you stop making yourself wrong, your energy is freed up. You are no longer stuck. You can sail on much easier. Don't stop for long at anger, though. Keep moving! Celebrate every bit of progress, awareness, and happiness.

Soothe yourself.
You are where you are, and now you know how to move!

I'm Not Resistant!

NO ONE INTENDS to be resistant, have a low vibration, or be unhappy. If you are still unhappy and your life is not working as well as you'd like, even after reading this book, you've only just begun. Read it again. Take an Online Course and get more immersed in it.

Here's a follow-up letter I wrote to students after a Five-Day Retreat: "People who have difficulty allowing feeling may struggle longer. Because they've resisted feeling for so long, huge amounts of emotion try to rise, and it scares them. It's astonishing to find that feeling is one of the most feared experiences on the planet.

One participant experienced the full power of his God Self during the initiation in the Five-Day Retreat. He felt he was about to levitate as he stood there, basking in the energy. Then a few days later he had a *huge* movement of old, stagnant energy (fear, terror, sadness, grief) accompanied by intense physical symptoms. Having relied on "human strength and mind over matter" for more than thirty-five years, he didn't realize how much he had resisted feeling. He'd been doing Divine Openings, while resisting it, for two years—a superhuman feat! Holding back from anything takes a tremendous amount of your energy. That's why he'd felt so tired in the retreat.

The eventual and inevitable awakening of the True Self within pushes out anything that is not in alignment with it. Bliss tends to bring up its opposite and push out anything that is not bliss. Then that lower feeling rises. That's part of bringing your enlightenment down to Earth, and becoming fully embodied. That may take a while, but it really doesn't have to. Men sometimes have more difficulty with feeling deeply, having been trained their whole lives not to show "weakness." What a handicap, having much of one's own Instrument Panel be off limits! For a man, anger might be OK, where sadness or tears are not allowed. For women, anger is often taboo, where tears are permissible.

A war hero who fears no gun, bomb, or knife might break down into a twitching, terrified heap when confronted with his own feelings or the illness of a parent or child. That feeling can't be shot, stabbed, or conquered, but resisting it only causes suffering.

Being around me is intense. There's a powerful, accelerated, evolution-inducing vortex that causes energy and feelings to move. I love it, but some romantic and work partners who were in strong resistance and didn't wish to feel and evolve simply couldn't remain in this field of resonance. Some actually melted down and had to go away.

Sometimes people attempt to manage everything with the mind to avoid feeling. They try to *think through feelings,* which is a spiritual bypass. One man who is very, very powerful and successful in the business world had already admitted that feeling was his Waterloo. He fled one of my courses in cold sweats with his back muscles completely seized up. That is how terrifying it can be for some people to feel when the mind has told them for decades, "You must not feel THAT! Anything but that!" I know he will complete the course when he's ready—in the meantime he's in the online courses giving himself time to soften into feeling. He's a lovely, generous, sensitive person. He wants to make a difference, and does. He's shared Divine Openings with his whole family.

Once we soften around any challenge, Grace moves us, guides us, helps us very quickly. People who commit and let go do not have big difficulties—Grace gives you a sweet, easy, lovely unfolding. But you need to know what can happen if resistance is strong. You're not losing your mind, and you're not dying. (Some medical alarms do need attention.) Soften and give it over to The Presence. It is truly not your job to do it alone."

Let it be easy. You get no extra points for doing it the hard way.

Be assured that Divine Openings doesn't make you feel anything that wasn't already there. It doesn't create a problem that didn't already exist. It only makes you aware of it so that it can move. While many of you are noticing big shifts by now, here's more help for how to let go.

Here are some clues that you might be unconsciously "prohibiting feeling":

- You analyze, rationalize, or think everything through instead of feeling it through.

- You get blindsided and surprised by people and events. You couldn't feel your Instrument Panel readings and didn't feel it coming.

- You're always in a hurry, rarely sit still, and stay constantly busy.

- Or you have low energy and don't get much done. You're tired, heavy, and weary a lot from holding back all that feeling that wants to move. Your metabolism is slow.

- Numbness. You're not sure what you feel on some subjects. Body sensation is muffled.

- You talk a lot. Talking is addictive for you.

- You have to be with people all the time, and can't be happy alone.

- Or you avoid people or intimacy and have shallow relationships.

- You're always cheerful, but things don't go well. If so, the cheer doesn't match the vibration you're actually feeling.

- You suspect you have blind spots—vibrations you're unaware of—things happen and you don't know how you created them.

- You're cynical or resigned, or you settle for less than you really want.

- You act tough and you attract tough treatment by other people and by life.

- Or you get more "spiritual," and try to go around the feelings with positive thinking, meditation, spiritual bypass, or other means.

What if after reading the above list, you suspect you're not feeling as much as you could? Don't judge yourself—you got trained not to feel. It's not your fault. Be incredibly kind to yourself. Treat yourself like a sweet, precious newborn. You take care of your car, your home, your kids, friends, and pets. Now, how about yourself?

Do the Daily Pleasure Practices and Thirty Ways To Raise Your Altitude from the end of the book. Take an online course, watch the videos, and listen to the audios to immerse yourself in this higher vibration. Demonstrate your intentions and commitments to yourself with action. Ask to feel. Then be willing to feel. I'm always astounded to hear how many people listen to my audios every day—it helps them keep their vibration rising and their mind occupied with positive input.

You're going to be fine now. Divine Openings makes life easier pretty quickly, and the fun starts. Still, some people find they need more help to break through deep numbness, strong resistance, blind spots, or over-analytical minds. Let in the support you need. See the resources at the back of the book. So many tell us they appreciate that we don't drop them flat after this book.

Questions People Ask

I'm afraid I'll become addicted to this. The reason 12-step programs work so well is that they show you that all addictions are just a misdirected search for spiritual bliss. If you get addicted to you Large Self, that's the real thing—it's healthy like being addicted to good food. You can go inward, get quiet and experience this energy anytime. You don't need a Divine Opening to get there once you've found that relationship within, so you won't get dependent on us. Keep coming for vibrational support until you don't need it. Then you might just stay connected for community with people who get your reality.

I can't just become enlightened without doing the hard work on myself to get through my own fears, beliefs, and blocks. Yes, you can. Do the practices, let go and receive the Grace. Let The Divine do the heavy lifting. That it has to be hard is the *old paradigm.* If Divine Openings ever starts to feel like hard work, you've dragged the "toil on the old spiritual path" paradigm into it. You can let that go now.

I wonder if this first time experience was the biggest high I will ever get, and will I be disappointed in future Divine Openings. Every experience will be different, yes. It will ebb and flow like the tides. It is cumulative, and does grow deeper over time. You cannot predict when the peak experiences, the cosmic experiences, bliss, or laughter will come. Enjoy each for what it is, don't hang on, let them go.

How can I feel better when this moment sucks? Well, my dear, it is your response to this moment that creates your tomorrow. You simply cannot afford to focus for too long on what you don't want, what went wrong, or how awful it is. Sure, you are "justified" in your attitude; everyone will validate you. But the cost of dwelling in that justified victimhood is *just too high.* Don't let circumstances and people be your "excuse" for staying down, and not aligned with your Large Self. Pivot your thoughts from what went wrong to what you want, over and over. Or Dive In until it rises. Choose power over powerlessness. Choose happiness over being right.

How do people get good things when they don't appear to be feeling good? He's mean to his employees, he has a great girlfriend, and he's rich! It isn't fair! Well-being and abundant flow is the natural state of the universe. God loves all of you. Good things are always flowing to you and everyone else, without judgment, from God's Grace. Somehow that guy is letting that good in. Even when your altitude is low, God looks for every little crack of least resistance, every opportunity to give you your good. Judging closes down your pipes so it can't get to you as easily, not because you're "bad," but because your Large Self doesn't judge, so you're out of alignment with your Large Self. If you're in victim mode, resenting, or judging, you're not in receiving mode.

You can never know how that guy feels inside. Pay attention to how *you* feel. Look at your *own* Instrument Panel—that you can know. It's not so much that you need to work to create more of what you want; you just need to stop resisting the flow of good, the dominant energy of the universe. You can let it in or resist it. Get out of the way! Forget about trying to figure out why people you judge as bad have the goodies. You can't read their Altimeter, and *it's none of your business!* You can't feel what's inside them and know what they're thinking and vibrating; it's "relative," it doesn't always show on the outside, and their words and actions don't tell the whole story. They can sound grumpy but have a great money vibration. You can look and talk positive and seem spiritual and yet have a terrible money or love vibration.

Judging people who have money and success for how they use it lowers *your* altitude and slows you down. Envy is a low vibration that shrinks your pipes and slows the flow of good to you. Just focus on your own vibration. Mind your own business.

Sleep

THE PRESENCE is always looking for an opening to give you more. The Divine even uses your sleep time to bring you what you need, since during sleep you leave physical density behind, open, and relax into non-resistance. You refresh and recharge in the pure positive energy of the Non-Physical. Grace and rejuvenation is allowed into your life as you sleep because your mind is out of the way—there's no resistance. That's why you feel so good after sleep or meditation.

Notice this tomorrow morning: you always feel good when you first wake up. But if your normal daytime vibrational set point is lower than your Large Self's, you'll feel less good milliseconds *after* waking as you slide from non-resistance back down to your lower set point. If this happens, do a pleasurable Divine Openings practice each morning to raise it before beginning your day. Breathe deeply for five minutes with a tiny smile on your lips.

You usually feel better and circumstances improve after resting or the pleasure practices at the end of the book. Give yourself plenty of them every day. You're always thinking and doing something anyway, so it might as well be something that feels good!

Life is on your side. Will you be on your side too?

When Will I Be Enlightened?

FOCUS ON the good things that have already happened. If you "work on" and focus on what's lacking, you'll create more of it. Focus on the fact that your Large Self is already "there," and that it calls to you constantly, and doesn't judge how long it takes or if you stray. Experience the *perfect imperfection* that you already are.

As the Divine Openings unfold for you, you might experience increased bliss, love, causeless laughter or any emotion. You might have improvements in work or money, attitude shifts, a breakthrough in a relationship, increased or decreased energy (temporarily), sleep changes, quieter mind (or temporarily busier mind.) You might notice tingling, physical sensations, physical detox, new inspirations, boredom, or temporary emptiness.

The best news, in any case, is there's nothing to do or work on. Even contrast propels you. Lightly, briefly witnessing what you're feeling causes energy to move. You see, when you did clearing or "healing work" habitually, it just created more of what you were looking to clear or heal. Now it's moving and rising spontaneously, as energy is supposed to move. Your Divine Intelligence orchestrates it, and hard work is over. You can let go of the old paradigm of working on yourself now.

Appreciation smooths your progress. Say, "thank you for showing me what I'm vibrating." "Thank you for moving the old out of my life so there's room for the new to come in." "I appreciate what every contrast shows me. Now what's next?" "I'm curious and excited about what's coming!"

The more you focus on what is not here, the more you delay it. The more you stress about your enlightenment, the slower it comes. Relax and enjoy the ride, and better things *flow to you*. Above all, it's all about joy. There's really nowhere to get *to*.

Start focusing more on how you feel right now, and less on outcomes.

In general, this massive realignment process goes like this: you receive a Divine Opening and directly experience the Divine in you. Then it begins to work on you from the inside out. The pure positive bliss energy you feel might also stir up slow and dense energies that are clogging the pipes. You may feel it as it moves up the scale—you may not. Then love and joy can flow through the pipes better than ever. You may go up and down for a while, and then you stabilize at a higher level. Then you go higher in another cycle, and stabilize there.

Increasingly you feel happy even when there's no "reason" to, or love where there was none. Eventually, nothing can get you down for long.

It may feel like you're unhooking from the matrix, seeing behind the curtain, as you remember who you really are. The territory is unfamiliar, and it puts us all outside our comfort zones, but the help is there within and without. Increasingly, we can relax and let the Flow of Life show us where to go and how to get there. The "softer" we are and the more we let go, the easier it is.

I had imagined awakening would be some ethereal state where mystical visions appeared, and all my challenges stopped. There are fewer challenges. Challenges still occur, but there is more ease, and even relish, in handling them. It's a creative game. We came here to have a variety of experiences and contrasts. The contrasts are less extreme, but they are still there. They help us know even more clearly what we want. Eating the "fruit of the tree of the knowledge of good and evil" represents to me the birth of rational thinking, polarities and contrasts, and the Free Will choice to choose between the contrasts. In any given moment we can either align with The Divine in us or choose struggle. The choice is ours, but it's never final. You can re-choose.

Life has indeed become magical and full of synchronicity and ease, yet I, and others in this process, find it subtle most of the time. It's more like a steady stream of "all is well," a smooth unfolding of daily life that hums along without drama, punctuated with joy and occasional bursts of causeless bliss.

Human neurology is not yet evolved to handle the extreme voltage of pure Divine Bliss all the time. It ebbs and flows. Surf it!

I promise you this—it will still feel bad to slip down into the lower vibrations. It is supposed to! When you're not aligned with your Large Self, it is supposed to feel bad so you'll go back up. Dropping just a bit might even feel as bad as being at the bottom used to feel.

During my twenty-one days of silence, my Honeymoon With The Divine, I asked for a love like I'd never had—the compatible, co-creative, and passionate partnership I'd always wanted. Within a month of returning home, I met a lovely man so easily, so naturally, and it developed so smoothly and quickly that I marveled only upon looking back. I had thought fireworks would flare and trumpets would sound, but there was only the sound of our laughter, and a quiet peaceful flow of sweet casual experiences that seemed so inexplicably natural that I decided, "I think I'll keep doing this." It sure takes the pressure off both people to enjoy the moment and put aside the judgments of what it is supposed to be or where it's going. The voice inside had simple advice, "Enjoy!" That relationship was so much fun, and in some ways better than any before it, yet it was not forever. I enjoyed every minute of it and then let it go two years later when it was no longer a vibrational match. Some relationships have expiration dates, and there's nothing wrong with that.

The right people and things always appear at the right time, close on the heels of the need, or often even slightly before the need, in a way that serves everyone involved.

Within two years I went from no income to being prosperous. I'm not independently wealthy, but I'm "independently happy"—independent of outer conditions. Anything I need comes. There's been steady growth in Divine Openings each year, and I'm happy it wasn't faster so I didn't get overwhelmed and overworked. If anything, I'm still holding back a bit on growth to maintain balance. I'm not impatient, nor particularly ambitious—I do all this out of a natural enjoyment of the unfolding. Notoriety grows simply because I've helped a lot of people and they tell a lot of people.

Problems are fewer and fewer, and life isn't about problems anymore. Health has improved. I had forgotten about those health issues until just now, so it's fun to celebrate that. Energy has increased. It's a steady, upward path. The worries of past years are gone, and the occasional flicker of doubt quickly fades, either by itself, by diving into it for a few minutes, or by deliberately raising my altitude.

The mind still loves to make up scary stories. Even when you're free the mind might still say you're not. That's what that wrong-seeking missile of a mind does. I just don't believe everything I think anymore! I am keenly guided by the voice of my Large Self that sounds like me, only smarter. It is constant if I stay up there where I can hear it. *God doesn't go away, but sometimes we do!* We can always return to it.

My guidance is not usually a flashy thing—the mystical experiences were rare, but one day it was clear that something had clicked in. "I've got it." I know my power. I know from my Large Self perspective that all is well. I don't just believe it—I know it.

Enlightenment is just being in the Flow of Life.

Let Life Surprise You

TEARS FILLED MY EYES remembering how sixteen years before this book was written I set the intention to create Heaven on Earth. I was nowhere near it, and didn't have the slightest clue how to do it, or even an inkling of what it would be like. How many times had I despaired it would never happen? Only a few years before Divine Openings I learned to raise my altitude easily and consistently—then Divine Openings continued to raise it until it was un-crashable. But this stage is only the beginning. Once you get to a high cruising altitude, the journey really gets exciting.

Sometimes I set a destination and go there, but usually I let Life surprise me: as with this book being read in over 140 countries, having a worldwide website, photographing covers for a holistic magazine and writing articles for it for a while, writing a theme song for a film, writing, singing, and recording my own original music, having five books and twenty one online courses, giving retreats in Europe, most of it without planning, intending, or striving. The lack of attachment to specific outcomes and the willingness to be surprised helps a lot—*things go great in my absence.*

Miracles are normal when you're in the flow of life—when they're not happening, that is not normal. Deep appreciation brings even more of it, so stop and rave often.

You become accustomed to each high you reach until it becomes quite normal for you, even a plateau of sorts. Then you reach for another plateau, thrill in it, and then it becomes normal. The universe expands as you expand.

Waves of ecstasy might wash through your body during mundane activities. One day my truck wouldn't start, and there was absolutely no dip in my mood, only a tiny sense of inconvenience as I decided what to do, made a plan, and carried it out. The next day as I rode with the tow truck driver to the repair place I had chosen, I suddenly began to experience an almost orgasmic full body ecstasy for absolutely no reason. It was inexplicable by all logical standards. My truck was broken, I knew it was going to cost me time and money, and there I was in bliss, talking with the driver, enjoying a raging, passionately physical sense of being alive—life force flowing through my body, lighting up every cell.

I want to relate a rather mundane sequence of events that followed that magical experience. You might think God has better things to do than take care of our ordinary needs, but throughout the next month, I was reminded that The Indweller cares about our every want.

Once the mechanic checked the truck, I got some unwelcome news—the warranty did not cover that particular issue, and the bill was for hundreds of dollars I had planned to use for something more fun. I used to call that "bad news," but now I'm pretty clear that there isn't any such thing. These days, even as I hear the "bad news," I think something like, "Well, that was unexpected… hmmm." I did have a momentary dip, but within an hour I had rebounded and determined to simply let in more money fast, which happened in the next week. The choice was simple: feel bad, point the nose of the plane downward, and create more unpleasant and costly incidents, or decide to raise my vibration, feel good, and point the nose of the plane upward, and change trajectory. That's an easy decision, isn't it? It worked, and any upset faded within hours. That's my mantra now: "Is pointing the nose down, no matter how justified I might be, worth it? Is it going to help create what I want?"

Days later, I decided it was time to purchase a new truck but quickly found that the trade-in value of my old truck was far less than I had thought. I'd have to sell it myself—not something I wanted to take the time to do. I was definitely ready for a change, a fresh set of wheels that matched my new vibration. I simply shrugged, stayed focused on what I wanted, and walked out thinking, "Oh well, I wonder what will happen to solve this?" Within hours a friend offered to buy the truck for what I owed, and was delighted at the price. I sold it to him, and strolled back into the dealership ready to buy my new truck within two days.

In another surprise twist, the truck I had wanted was already sold. Again, not what I expected. I was immediately sure it was for the best, and sure enough, I found out I had been spared a mistake. The salesman had been wrong about the towing capacity, and it would not have pulled my horse trailer well. I proceeded to shop for another two weeks, walking car lots, comparing gas mileage and towing capacity stats, dodging salespeople's manipulations. I kept changing my mind, thinking, "Should I get a car, or a truck that will pull my horse trailer? Or get both?" I went back and forth, got myself confused, became too mental and analytical about it, and lost the flow. One day out in the hundred-degree heat at noon walking a car lot, and feeling light-headed, I said to myself, "I'm working way too hard at this. This is so unlike my normal life these days to work this hard at anything. I need to get clear on what I want. I'll go home and relax." I went home and rested, going to bed early from the heat exhaustion. Then my partner decided to buy a truck—so I could pull the trailer without buying a truck.

The new day dawned with a fresh new feeling, and the next night I spontaneously decided to stop off at a car lot just after closing, on my way home, and walked among the cars in a light carefree mood, caressed by a cool breeze. My gaze fell upon a deep metallic red convertible. My heart leaped for joy. It felt good. Suddenly, it was clear—the vehicles I'd been telling myself I should get were boring, and that was the reason I had not been able to make up my mind. In my heart of hearts I didn't really like any of them! This car *felt* good.

From out of a closed showroom, a salesman appeared, and I drove the car, thrilling at the fresh air and the open sky. I had wanted one of these convertibles, this exact model, for years. The salesman said the car had just come in yesterday. The reason I hadn't found it earlier was it wasn't there yet, and I was stuck on the truck idea. All my focused "working" had kept me from seeing something different than I had expected. I use this mundane example of a car, but how often do we "miss seeing it" in business, in relationship, in other areas of life?

I laugh as I think of this sequence of events—how "lightening up" on the search and loosening the grip had made me happy even before the solution occurred. This moment is all there ever is, after all, and straining forward into some future moment is a recipe for unhappiness. It's all about joy after all. It wasn't the car that made me happy—getting happy allowed the car to come to me. The car was just a byproduct of the happiness, a small material expression of that happy energy.

The car story illustrates that The Presence cares about every detail of our lives, just like a best friend does. Cars are trivial in my world; I don't care what people think about what I drive or what status it confers. It just has to feel good *to me*. Feeling good is such an important indicator to me—when something feels good I know I'm in the flow. The Presence wanted me to feel good and have fun driving my car—wanted me to have something that I had not let myself have for many years. Our Large Self doesn't judge what we want; it just delivers it. A friend joked, "When you go around all the time with your crown chakra open, you want a convertible car that matches." Driving along on a cool evening, I'd look up at the miracle of the starry sky, and appreciate my Large Self. Appreciation is the single best way to elevate your joy instantly.

Day to day, it may seem not much is changing, but you'll look back in six months, and it will be clear how much has changed. Changes in your life might be subtle or dramatic, but you're moving, and movement feels good. By setting simple intentions but not gripping on them, forces are set in motion to shift things *for you*. One year into Divine Openings my work had shifted from local private sessions and classes to a worldwide audience, retreats, and online courses without working hard at all.

Expanding the Universe

LOOK AT ALL the things you think you need to do, be, and have—from a fine home, to education, to achieving enlightenment, to being in love, to serving others. You want all that because you think you will be happier by being, doing, or having it. See if you can think of one single thing you want that doesn't hold the promise of making you feel better—better about yourself, your loved ones, or the condition of humanity. So, here's the secret: get happy now, before you get the job or the mate, before you are enlightened, before you become who you want to be, before all wars end, before politicians tell the truth, before your mother changes, before you get rich and skinny. Then you have what you really wanted in the first place—and you have it right NOW. Then you lift all of humanity too.

The secret to happiness is to savor the waiting between the time you decide what you want and the day it arrives on the physical plane. You desire it, your Large Self creates it on the spot, indeed "becomes it," and starts the party. Your job is to let go, relax, release tension and resistance, and get your altitude up, so you're vibrating in alignment with your Large Self about it. You get yourself to the party, and you're the last key piece. Then the party appears on the physical plane.

You will always and forever be in that gap between your next desire and the physical arrival of it, because as each dream is fulfilled, you will dream up another one immediately. That is your creative, ever-expanding nature. Get used to being eternally, happily "on the way to _____."

"Wanting" keeps life flowing through you. You'll either savor the waiting and be happy now, even though the next dream is not yet here, or you will always be suffering because the next dream is not yet here. Which one feels better? Which one speeds up the arrival of your desires and which one slows them down?

Savor the waiting. Enjoy the journey. That journey turns out to be your life.

At a more advanced stage, you'll notice that the biggest thrill isn't the physical manifestation of something; the biggest thrill comes in that (now!) moment that your spirit begins to soar as you feel it forming in the Non-Physical. You birth an intention, and you feel the universe becoming pregnant with your creation, *and you revel in that feeling* before it ever shows up.

With your heightened senses you feel the energy as it lines up, you hop on that wave of your creation like a surfer, and you surf the pure energy of it while it's still in the Non-Physical. That Non-Physical swelling is as pleasurable as the physical outcome, much as a pregnant woman feels and loves her baby before she ever sees it. The universe enjoys the expansion you created whether you let it into your personal physical world or not, but of course you're letting it in now. Are you beginning to really get who and what you are?

You expand the universe *by creating what you want.*

When your heart leaps, your soul sings, and life looks brighter—in that moment you're happy whether that manifestation ever shows up or not. Paradoxically, that's when the manifestation you so long wanted can most easily come—the job, the car, the lover, the bliss, or the enlightenment. It will seem matter of fact to you by the time it comes. "Why, of course it's here, I've been surfing on the wave of it. I didn't have to wait for it to get happy. *I took the shortcut* to happiness."

Feeling good has become such a strong habit that family dramas, even my father's life-threatening illnesses, didn't sink me. Small dips, perhaps. Usually not even that. I am now like a boat that bobs to the surface no matter how many waves crash over that boat. I try to enjoy the rocking. This is contagious and it has buoyed up my friends and family many times in the face of serious difficulties. By being who you are, and creating the feelings and manifestations you create, you add to the universe, which expands it. Your happiness is felt, as a tangible atmosphere, like weather, across the universe. Really.

I'm not floating above it all, nor jaded or detached. Far from it. I am solidly grounded in my body sensations and emotions, and life is more intensely felt than ever—I just feel higher vibrations more often, and stay in the lower vibrations less. The norm is a smooth hum. I still have frequent, intense surprise attacks of sweet wonder and awe, tears stream down my face from the sweetness of a simple hug, every cell in my body feeling as if it could burst from the fullness. And that comes and goes like all feelings and experiences do. There is no way to hold onto it. Life moves. Energy wants to move. Let it move.

Divine Opening

SOFTLY CONTEMPLATE the work of art for two minutes, then close your eyes and allow your experience for fifteen or more minutes. Appreciate your opening.

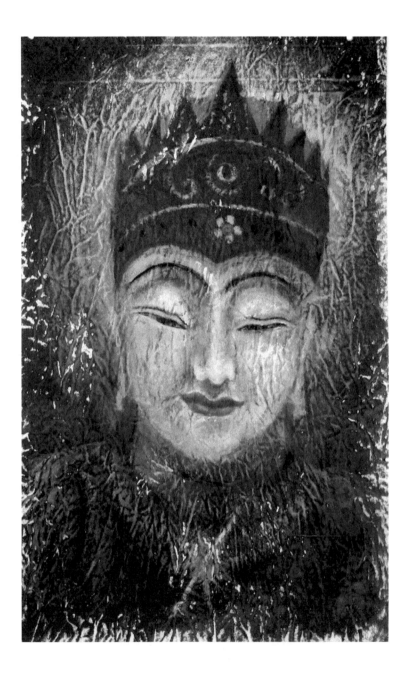

Figure 9—Thai Goddess, a painting by Lola Jones

If Your Bliss Seems To Fade

SOME SAY after a time, "My high has worn off." But when I ask them to look at it, they see it hasn't actually faded at all; they are higher overall than ever, but the initial newness and thrill is now taken for granted. And now their Large Self is calling them higher, so they feel the newly opened gap between where they are now and where their Large Self is calling them to expand. While seeking is over with Divine Openings, the expansion is endless.

This true story says it quite entertainingly. A friend took a course from me years ago, before Divine Openings. She was on food stamps, lived in a tiny rental cottage, and was depressed. After the course, she was renewed, and soon started a company that became successful worldwide.

Then she read this book and came to a Divine Openings event years later and said she was stuck. She said, "I'm right back where I was ten years ago before I took your other course! I'm single and in debt, and I'm not happy about it." I looked around the room and everyone was buying that story. I laughed and said, "Darlin', that is what the mind does to you. I beg to differ with this dire assessment. I know a bit about your life. You are vastly beyond where you were ten years ago. You are not on food stamps. You have a successful company. You own a home and horses. You travel constantly. You were just on Oprah. You got used to your new success level and now you want more. You are merely on a plateau, complaining, which prevents your next expansion. You're a creative being. You want to stretch your wings further and fly higher. You came to the right place— again!"

She grinned sheepishly, then laughed. Our wrong-seeking-missile-mind can take the small-self perspective and tell the worst possible story about *any situation*. It ignores all the good and goes straight for what is wrong. It discounts our progress and pounces on what hasn't happened yet.

Experience is relative. When you fall in love with someone new, it's a rush of new feelings and sensations. Then as you are together longer, you may actually love them more deeply, but the thrilling before-and-after contrast isn't there anymore. As the relationship matures the love is actually stronger and more real. Divine Openings is like that. Humans perceive, feel, and even appreciate *contrast and drama* more than *sameness*, and any exciting feeling eventually becomes "normal" to you. Keep it fresh and alive and growing by raving every day about how great it is. If you complain that the thrill is gone, it will indeed be gone, by your word.

With Divine Openings, it's as if you've met and fallen in love with your Large Self, the larger part of you. It's a huge contrast from where you were, so the thrill is huge when you first feel it. It's the ultimate love affair. But you will become used to this new relationship, and even though it's always deepening, it will just feel normal. If you complain about the lack of excitement, you create more lack of it. If you constantly rave about what you have, you create more of it.

If you won the lottery, you'd jump up and down and scream, "I'm rich, I'm RICH!" But in a year you wouldn't still be doing that. Hopefully you'd appreciate it, but you would be used to it, calmer about it. You'd even begin to take it for granted. And you'd soon want more in your life.

Enlightenment cannot and will not freeze your bliss into a static state that stays the same for ever after. That would be impossible. Energy wants to move, life is change, your Large Self wants you to expand and grow. Use your Free Will to create new joys and fresh highs rather than expecting the old ones to stay. You're happiest when you fly ever upward on the fresh thermals of your own heart's desires no matter how modest or grand they are. It's all relative. If you are one whose desires are big, whose thermals are fast and high, you will need a brisk pace of evolution to keep up with your dreams and stay fulfilled. If you've always been content with a modest life, modest movement will keep you happy. When you cling to what was good yesterday and don't allow yourself to go to the next level, you won't feel good. When it's time to release resistance and move—let go of the old, no matter how great it has been, and go for more!

If your bliss has faded, you're holding yourself back. It's supposed to feel bad, just like the red light on your car's Instrument Panel is supposed to tell you your emergency brake is on. It's supposed to feel bad to want something and not let yourself have it. It's supposed to feel bad when your Large Self is calling you to a party, and you're not letting yourself go. Appreciate the valuable information. Get yourself to the next party. Get a life. Or an expanded life.

Blocking yourself isn't good for you and it's supposed to feel bad. Don't wait for life to mirror it to you in the form of accidents, unwanted events, emotional stress, disease, or pain in your body. Allow movement!

Resistance feels bad. Letting go feels good. Your Instrument Panel works!

What To Do If:

1. The small self grabs the controls, you get hung up in small-self concerns, being right, working too hard, or anything low on the emotional scale. Your Instrument Panel will read a lower altitude, and it's supposed to feel bad, so you'll notice! Check who's driving, and tip the nose up, or Dive In. Use the *Thirty Ways To Raise Your Altitude* at the end of the book.

2. Your thoughts are in control. When you choose your thoughts and feelings you can keep your altitude up consistently. If you let stories take over, go on autopilot, and let circumstances, other people, or the outer world lead, your altitude will drop. *Choose!* Choose alignment with your Large Self. Then you don't have to specify the details of what you want; let it come in the perfect form for you. Co-creation is a two-way street. Sometimes you deliberately decide what you want, sometimes you put it on the God List, let go, and be surprised.

3. You let outside forces bring you down. Soften and allow your feelings about those things you can't change—it's the opposite of resistance and you'll be surprised how much and how quickly it helps. Hold your own center. Focus inward, not outward. Stop watching TV and reading bad news. All is well within. There is an un-shakable peace there, as at the eye of the hurricane, where your Large Self always lives.

4. An emotion wants to move, and you resist. The emotion or the resistance may be unconscious. You don't have to go digging for the problem. Just look at your life. There will be clues. Example: People are being combative with you. Look at your life and notice any grudge you've been holding against someone, or negative thoughts about something. That's attracting aggression. That is your cue to soften and Dive In. Or suddenly, you'll see a belief that is holding you back. Relax, tip the nose up, and what you need to know comes to you.

5. **You are holding back from being who you really are.** Life is calling you to the party and you're not letting yourself go. You know it's time for a new job, vacation, next level relationship, to write your book, perform your music, or come out of the closet, but you may have very logical reasons *(excuses!)* why you can't: "I have responsibilities, it won't work, can't afford it, can't face it, I owe it to (someone) to be who I am not." First soften around the feelings. It will free you up to move! Let go and let The Divine do the heavy lifting.

6. **You have tipped the nose of your plane down.** You are focusing on what's wrong in your life, in the world, or on what isn't here yet. That tips the nose downward. Instead, focus passionately and rave about what *is* right, what *is* here and what you *do* appreciate. You create your world out of thin air, out of nothing, from the Fertile Void. What feelings and experiences are you generating with your focus? What world are you creating? Focus on what you want, which will flow the energy in an upward direction, and tip the nose up. Soothe yourself now.

7. **Things aren't going well, yet you're unaware of your resistance.** Don't stay stuck. This is your LIFE! Take an online course or webinar series, come to a retreat, or get a session with a Divine Openings Guide.

Check your Instrument Panel. Where are you? When you're in the lower half of it, there is resistance involved. Don't go digging for dirt; that's not necessary or productive. Observe your life. Feel and flow. Let go, ask The Divine to do the heavy lifting, and you will go higher than before. There is nothing more important than your happiness, and your life is too important to let anything hold you back.

Nothing is more important than your vibration. It creates your reality.

More Ways To Realign With Your Large Self and Reclaim Your Happiness

1. Rave and appreciate. This is the most powerful thing you can do daily.

2. Soothe yourself. Talk to yourself like you would talk to a dear friend or child. Chat with The Presence, then answer yourself *as your Large Self.* This is a real dialog that builds over time.

3. Softly embrace where you are. Where you are is where you are, and where else could you be? Experience where you are fully. Give it over to The Divine. It will shift faster without resistance or judgment. Deep within you, all is well *right now.* Go within and feel it for yourself.

4. Accept that your Large Self is always ahead of you. Put all the things you want on the God List and let them go. Enjoy the journey, savoring each step. Soothe yourself with, "I'll get there. And then I'll want more. Enjoy now…. now…. and now."

5. Have regular "Dates with The Divine" and renew your romance with your Large Self. Go into the silence alone for a day without television, radio, email, phones or books. Speak to no one, and put all your focus on The Presence within. Talk only to The Presence and deepen your relationship. Talk, chat, laugh, cry, share, and appreciate. Nothing compares with that deep, sweet communion.

6. Move to uplifting music. Physical movement and play blasts you upward in vibration. The *Watch*

Where You Point That Thing music download comes with a movement video that's all about joy.

7. Remember who you are. You are a Divine being in a physical body. You chose to come here and experience contrasts, choose among choices, and co-create with The Creator.

8. Meditate regularly, even if for only ten minutes. It focuses you on what is real—the inner you, your Larger Self. Divine Openings has opened up your ability to meditate more deeply than ever before. Don't do it to "work on yourself" but to feel good. *Meditate for pleasure.*

9. Breathe for pleasure. Breathe in and out gently and naturally as you focus on your breath and body. Let your spine undulate with the breath. Relax. Don't work. Think soft. Emotions might arise and move. If they do, relish them. Be with them until they move up. Sometimes you can get to bliss. If you're over-revved or can't sleep, don't resist or make it wrong—breathe for pleasure. Lie there and soothe yourself, and you'll arise refreshed even if you don't sleep. Enjoy!

You'll begin to feel peace or bliss again as soon as you take one step, tip the nose up slightly, and deliberately soar upward. Bliss is the natural result of soaring on the flow of Life. The moment your energy stops flowing freely, or even slows down, you feel less good. There's a longer list of easy practices at the end of the book. Play at it—don't work at it!

Happiness is your natural state. Releasing resistance returns you to it.

Whether a heart's desire feels thwarted, or your plane's nose has drifted downward, your bliss will fade as the vibration drops and gets denser! Your Large Self is always moving and expanding, flying along on the current of *your desires*—it's not resisting at all. It's already at the party. Your party. Not allowing yourself to go there too will feel bad, *and it's supposed to.*

You must expand and flow with the current of Life in order to feel good again. That means allowing it all, wherever you are on the Instrument Panel. That means following your heart, whatever it wants. That means sometimes ignoring your mind, its limits, and whoever or whatever says you can't.

Let go to the flow. It might mean moving to Denmark, or it might be as simple as doing something mundane in your own back yard that makes your heart sing. It doesn't have to be big. When I want to go thrift store shopping, I go. It relaxes me, and for some odd reason, makes my heart soar. I can afford brand new clothes, but that doesn't give me the same zing. Go figure. I often visualize what I want to find there, and there's a big sense of adventure and wonder at where I'll find it, and how soon. Sometimes it's the same day. The important thing is to do it simply because it feels good.

Your Instrument Panel always tells you when it's time to expand. First you notice a subtle nudge from your Large Self—a thought or a desire. If you go with it, there's ease. If you ignore it, you'll slide down the Instrument Panel. If you ignore that, the message escalates, and you might experience physical symptoms like tension or stiffness or pain. If you ignore the subtle physical signals, illness could occur. It's a progressive system where your Instrument Panel flashes increasingly brighter warning lights and blares louder buzzers to tell you you're resisting.

While teaching a Divine Openings Course years ago, it became clear: I realized that like some of the students that day, I was still buying into the consensus reality that "work is hard" and "money is hard," thought forms that are completely pervasive in our scarcity-riddled world. I had begun to pick up a little stress, which is just information, a signal to *move, expand, let go*!

I decided (*intention* is all it takes at this stage) to create even more ease for myself. Each time we *intend*, new avenues open up, and new possibilities are magnetized to help us. In the seminar we all dived into the vibration that lies at the heart of the feeling that work is hard and money is scarce. It rose in vibration, and we were soon giggling at that absurd old notion. A new lightness came over us.

Releasing resistance by fully feeling through it restored my high. Then that momentum brought even more progress. In this new consciousness, the next day a new chain of events began unfolding effortlessly. First I got depressed! Of course, my mind protested, "This isn't progress! I'm going backwards. I don't get depressed anymore. Shouldn't I be immune from this by now?" But my Large Self gave me a quiet soothing feeling, assurance that this was perfect and if I didn't resist it would pass quickly. Resistance to feeling creates suffering.

I sat on the porch on a perfect day and dived into the vibration that felt like "depression," sensing that this was very old energy. I began to feel lighter and lighter and soon lost interest in the exercise, which is usually your cue that you are done with Diving In. I brought my laptop out to write, and soon, with no effort, I felt better than I had in weeks—it was a new high.

There was a domino effect as more guidance came in—I had a very subtle and easy urge to skip the glass of wine with dinner. A glass of wine occasionally is fine, but I felt a desire to get even more sparkling clear, and to maximize this new rise in altitude.

For many, alcohol gives that permission to feel extra good, as if somehow it's "not your doing." But you can feel good without any reason, and it's okay! I have a drink occasionally, but I love natural highs, and I'm so accustomed to being high that the substances and activities many people use to get high are actually a downward move for me. It's all relative.

The result of following this inwardly guided trail of mundane changes was that more money began to flow in with less work. I didn't analyze. I just felt and followed.

Notice that I don't often use euphemisms like abundance and prosperity. Many spiritual people use those fluffy words because they have judgments about *money* and can't bring themselves to say *"I want money."* So, check in: can you say, "I want cash"? Abundance and prosperity aren't accepted as legal tender and won't pay for groceries or rent. Money will.

The big message is to follow your urges and pay attention to how you feel. All else will come.

Feel and follow.

Pleasure Practices

THE UPWARD MOMENTUM continued, and I soon felt a whole new spontaneous level of permission to feel good. Most of us have some cultural or generational taboos, or self-imposed limits we don't know we have. We bought into "unquestioned assumptions" because everyone else believed it, and then it became part of the background of life, like the air you never notice you're breathing. Growing up, we pick up from the culture and the adults around us that we shouldn't feel *too* good, be too boisterous, enjoy our body or sex too much, receive too much money, or have it too easy. We were told desire is bad. We should work hard and not be "lazy" or decadent.

Somehow, that Puritan ethic had sneaked in and put some limits on my newly found pleasure. I could feel resistance in my body, especially tension in my neck! Suddenly I witnessed it and popped out of it. Spontaneously, I began to do even more things that felt good; I would lie in bed in the mornings, at nap time, or at bedtime, and just luxuriate in the softness of the sheets, enjoy the sensations on the skin, smile at the many things there are to appreciate about a simple bed. I'd snuggle my cheek on the pillow, and stretch out catlike in languorous delight at the sound of the wind in the trees. I took long hot baths with candles. I walked on my land, not for exercise this time, but for pleasure. Profound bliss came over me. Ahh, I had missed that feeling. It was like coming home. We love the game of getting lost and coming home as much as babies love peek-a-boo. We love the contrast of it.

Desire for expansion, for opening, and for more drives the universe. It doesn't have to be profound, or for a lofty purpose. Your "wanting" moves delightfully delicious energy through you, and that movement expands the universe because your Large Self runs ahead with it even if you never do it. Your fulfilling your desires forwards life in the universe even more. Feeds it. Expands it. Your joy sends out a ripple that lights up the universe. Your peace and joy are that important. You are that valuable.

Desire that feels like "craving what you can't have" actually hurts you. Craving for a partner, or money or success while feeling a gnawing lack of it your gut tips the nose down. Dive In until your desire feels good and full of possibility. Or give that subject a rest—things will go better in your absence.

If you want to make a difference in the world, be joyful. It makes you a broadcast tower radiating a vibrational message of love, joy, and power.

The greatest bliss always occurs at the point of a new energetic expansion.

One New Year's Eve, I had slept late, and I couldn't quite get my motor started. This was odd. I usually wake ready to go, go, go, powered by Source Energy. I even know how to generate energies when there aren't any (we do create it all.) After a great breakfast of pancakes and sausage, I got an inspiration to sit under a tree and do nothing. Energy began to return.

I fired up my John Deere garden tractor and mowed giant spirals in the tall yellow grass in the front pasture. I kept going for hours and mowed about four more acres just for fun, like a kid on a go-cart. Watching the land become manicured and beautiful gives me enormous satisfaction. I cannot describe to you the thrill I felt as the sun went down. It was ecstatic. I don't know why it feels so good to do those things, and I don't care. It doesn't matter why something feels good to you. It doesn't need to have a point, it doesn't even have to be productive, and no one else needs to understand it. Just do it. You're adding to the joy in the universe.

You may feel like you have "too much work to do" to allow yourself to do pure Pleasure Practices—things that are not income producing, or responsible, or on your to do list. But you must do the things your heart wants to do. Those things are literally food for your soul, and if you starve your soul, how can you really live, much less be productive? Since there is no deadline saying you must do your Pleasure Practices, your weeks can continue to fly by without ever doing them—unless you give yourself permission and carve out time for them.

What are Pleasure Practices for you? Painting a picture, gardening, having coffee with a friend, teaching the dog tricks, or playing with kids? Let your Large Self lead you in its mysterious ways.

That very night after the mowing, my energy and passion skyrocketed. I had some big inspirations that led to "productive action" in my work, and they were fun, outside the box ideas. I felt renewed and enthusiastic about going to a New Year's Eve party, where before I was ambivalent about whether to go out, and I met lots of interesting new people and had a great time. I met a woman who could help me with some technical challenges. Doing those simple heart's desires led me on a productive, upward path.

Let go of "shoulds" and judgments about being a realistic, responsible adult, and instead, do a Pleasure Practice at least once a day—if not five or six times. You'll be amazed at what happens in other areas of your life when you allow that flow. When people say they're working harder to make their business grow, I'll grin and say, "Take a vacation. Things will go great in your absence."

As I followed my feelings further, I realized I really wanted to stop doing so many private sessions and lead more courses instead. Within a month I was doing mostly courses. By the time I decided to create online classes, I realized three people who knew how to set that up had already showed up in my life. Soon I was helping ten times more people in one fifth of the time it used to take. Magic.

Do Pleasure Practices—things that feel good to you.

APPLY IT TO YOUR LIFE: List some Pleasure Practices for this week, just to feel good!

1.
2.
3.
4.
5.
6.
7.
8.
9.
10.

Now, what are you waiting for? Start doing them!

Dream Intentions

DREAM INTENTIONS (I used to call them dream assignments) are one of my favorite ways to create, since in dream state we have zero resistance. While asleep, we are fully open to our Large Self—set free from the density and limits inherent in human form. It's the least resistant we will ever be while in physical bodies. We revert to pure Non-Physical consciousness and rest, recharge, create, and play unfettered in the loving Presence of our Pure Divine Source.

I write down things my Large Self can take care of for me while I sleep, or just intend it as I drift off to Resistance-Free Land. After setting Dream Intentions, I let them go, breathing with a big sigh, "It's not my job. It's done." It's fun to create Dream Intentions with your partner.

It's like delegating upward to your Non-Physical team. Remember the idea of *bhakti paradina*, the God who is at your service? Think of it like your own personal team of managers and assistants who never sleep, know everything and everyone, and cheerfully work for you twenty-four hours a day, beyond time and space. Appreciate that the Larger You never sleeps, and can do anything. With Divine Openings, when you sleep, things go great in your absence. It's especially great now that life is about creating rather than just solving issues and problems—creating fun and adventure, designing your life however you want it. Do a quick check and notice which you're doing. Remember, you'll get what you expect!

You sleep better when you "give over" all your cares and concerns first. Go to sleep on a good note, and you rest better. Off-loading all your cares gives profound peace, releases resistance, and brings relief. If you're overwhelmed, make a list before bed, give it to The Divine, and let go. Inspiration will come later when you least expect it. Better yet, many things on the list just show up or get done without any effort. I like running across an old list—invariably, most of it is done—much of it without much effort from me. Or it never needed to be done. Something better came along that made it unnecessary.

"Bad" dreams with Divine Openings mean Grace is raising that lower vibration for you. There is nothing to analyze, do, or worry about. *It's not predicting anything bad.* Say soothingly to yourself, "It's being handled in my absence." Feel the feeling in your body—drop the story.

Dreams aren't just about solving problems; they're about cooking your desires and creations. I particularly like Dream Intentions when my desire is big, since my limiting thoughts and beliefs often can't fathom how it can happen. There are no limits in the Non-Physical, or in dreamland.

Divine timing may not agree with my timing, but if I give it over and wait, it always comes eventually, or something better happens. It's much better than wearing myself out trying to do it all myself, forcing my own timetable. So many things we think we have to do are just the mind's incessant nagging. They were never necessary, or wouldn't have worked anyway.

Remembering the dream or "getting the answer" is *not important*. You may remember nothing when you wake, yet the thing you asked for shows up spontaneously in synchronistic ways in good timing. Someone gives you a lead, a person or piece of information shows up, or an inspired idea enters your mind later when you least expect it. Dream Intentions are great for anything—business, money, personal, relationship, creative, and health—desires of any kind. How easy is that?

Dream on it.

Just Ask, Then Get Out of the Way!

WITH ALL OF these processes and techniques, we could forget the simplest and most powerful thing of all. Letting go and letting The Divine do the heavy lifting is always the most powerful thing you can do.

Talk to The Presence and chat about what you need and want. But don't keep *asking* over and over.

It's done. Asking repeatedly contradicts your desire and says, "I don't believe it's coming."

The party started when you asked. Focus on how you can get out of the way, release resistance, and get yourself to the party. For the simplest and most mundane needs, for realizing your dreams, communications with loved ones, business and money, relief of physical illness, the wisest decision, the best vacation plan, for humor and fun, The Presence knows what you want. Get yourself to the party.

The Presence is already there offering help in every moment, way before you ask, but your asking focuses *your* energy and aligns *you* with the solution. It reminds you to look for and let in the answers that are always being offered. It focuses you on getting to the party.

The most powerful thing you can ever do is give it over to The Presence, the Larger You.

How To Help Others

PEOPLE ASK how they can influence their families and co-workers to live an enlightened and happy life. Share this book with them. They'll pay more attention if you do your best to live it, while sharing your progress and imperfections with them. Being an example of it can mean saying, "Hey, I'm angry at you right now, so let's not talk until I have a chance to clean up my own feelings. I'm going for a walk to do just that. I'll be back. See you in a bit." Wow, what a powerful message! You're claiming your power instead of blaming them. This is a great way to teach kids to feel and be authentic, yet responsible.

You can roughly gauge your vibration by how much those around you are awakening. They'll mirror you to a great extent.

In an old relationship before Divine Openings, I kept wishing the man would do more personal development with me. Instead, he would continually bust me when I wasn't walking the talk, and he seemed to delight in doing things to get me to lose control of my emotions. Now I see he was not able to hear my wise words because my vibration and actions spoke louder.

You can only help people who are open to it. With friends and family, primarily intend to *allow them to be as they are, and manage your own feelings about it.* Dive In and lose any charge or attachment you have on their behavior first. Then you might say, "Ask if you want to hear my perspective," or "Would you like input, or are you just wanting me to listen?" When they express openness you can help, but when you give advice someone who doesn't want it, they might even feel made wrong or violated. How do you like it when someone tries to fix you?

Think about those cop movies: a crime is committed against one of the detective's family members, and he goes out to avenge the crime. His superior hears about it and tells him, "You're off the case! You're too emotionally attached!" He goes against orders and goes after the criminal, causing all kinds of havoc. You'll feel tension and chaos when you're not minding your own business.

When you're too attached, "take yourself off the case."

Our website makes it easy to share Divine Openings and leaves it to them. Share the web address with an open heart and let go of attachment to their response. You've done your part, and that feels good in itself.

There are moments when I realize a person cannot hear me from where they are. To them I must sound like I'm speaking in some foreign tongue. When they're complaining, suffering, and can't even see the possibility of a solution, I take a deep breath and say from the heart, "I hear you. It sounds tough." I stop talking, mind my own business, and walk the talk. It's their life, and pushing *too hard* to help is resistant and even controlling. Let others have their Free Will. They may surprise you and suddenly one day be open, or find a teacher they can hear better. There are different teachers for different people.

If you *are* called to counsel or teach formally, you may choose to train to become a Divine Openings Guide; then you can counsel and teach with great skill and effectiveness. Experienced school counselors and psychotherapists often become Guides to upgrade their skills to the leading edge, plus their work becomes less stressful. Doctors, lawyers, real estate agents, salespeople, entrepreneurs, and many other professionals become Guides so they can bring that extra magic and ease to their existing career.

Practice rather than preach. Help when it's appreciated.

Daydream For "Entertainment"

DAYDREAMS ARE FUN, and like meditation, are even more powerful than the relief from resistance you get at night, because you are consciously creating them. Exercising your focus as a conscious creator strengthens your power of intention, just as a muscle gains power from exercise.

There is no difference between a vivid daydream and reality, for the purposes of creating. Olympic athletes have used powerful visualization for years to improve their performance. Whenever you get a chance, daydream about what you want for yourself, and what you want to see in the world. That's all your Large Self sees anyway, all the time!

Daydreaming feels good because it aligns you with your Large Self. Your Large Self has already created that reality you want, and is just waiting for you to stop getting in the way and sending out resistant contradictory energy. It's waiting for you to get up to altitude with it so it can manifest in the physical. Best of all, it feels good right now!

You are not daydreaming to create something; it's already created. You were heard the first time you felt the desire, and your request was granted instantly. The party is happening in the Non-Physical realm right now, and it pops into the physical faster if you don't contradict and reverse it.

So often you're on the way to your desire, vibrating high about it, feeling great—then something in the outer world doesn't go like you expected, and you let your vibration go down. Now you're headed in the opposite direction of your desire. Don't let the outer world and its happenings influence you. Operate as if your vibration is the only thing that's important—because it *is* the only thing that matters ultimately. Anything happening in the outer world is temporary.

Daydreaming relaxes you so you don't contradict your desire with resistance, doubts, and slow down the manifestation. You daydream to get yourself to the party.

Daydreaming is a powerful way to savor the waiting and get out of the way.

Visualize mainly to keep yourself happy and out of the way.

Most of what we think, feel and vibrate was programmed and conditioned into us from birth. We got trained out of our natural Grace state. Much of our thoughts, feelings and the content of our current lives are not our own conscious creation, but more a mish-mash of hand-me-down ideas, beliefs, and thoughts from our family, society, and Ancient Mind. Now we get a fresh start.

Do your daydreaming for entertainment, and you will have the most relaxation and the least possible resistance on that subject. If you tell yourself it's for fun and not serious work, you'll relax, let go, and enjoy—and guess what? That's the very attitude that gets the fastest results.

Give yourself some "inner movie time." Add Technicolor sights, Dolby sound, smells, textures, dialogue and full-fledged feelings to your daydream script. Make it as real as you possibly can and stop if you lose the good feeling. Smile to yourself. Walk around in it rather than watching it. Add humorous scenes and you'll relax and release even more resistance. If you need help getting started, go test drive the car or horse you want, paint a picture, or cut out pictures and make a dream collage that gives you the *feeling* and the vibration you want.

One man set his table at meals with an extra plate *and food* for the ideal match who would soon show up in his life, and talked with her during meals, adding in what she might say too. Now, that is vibrating it right now. And yes, she did show up. An attorney daydreamed to lighten up before an upcoming hearing he was stressed about, and he smiled as he put humorous scenes in his movie. It worked. His hearing went smoothly. When you're relaxed, your power is freed up, and you'll perform miracles.

You're always "manifesting." You can't stop it.
You're just learning to do it deliberately rather than unconsciously.

APPLY IT TO YOUR LIFE: Try daydreaming right now. Pick something you'd love and dramatize it. Make it juicy enough that your mind assumes it's real. Feeling is more powerful than reading and thinking. Do this before you read on. Then plan one action or step to take toward your dream.

You can use daydreaming to help enlighten the world and create peace. First, get *yourself* there. You can do more good lying in your bed daydreaming what you want to see happening in the world than any legion of politicians, diplomats, missionaries, spiritual teachers, or soldiers can ever accomplish with action. So often, their tension and the "pushing against" actually creates more of the discord they are supposedly trying to eliminate. They get in discord within themselves. I rarely see a happy activist. Action doesn't produce results. Energy alignment produces results. Action just completes what was already done in the Non-Physical—but it often looks like it was the action that did it.

When this altruistic daydreaming practice feels good that tells you that you are in alignment with your Large Self. Simply lie relaxed and close your eyes. Create a daydream in which all is well, all is working out and everyone is prospering. As your power increases, you can offset thousands or even millions of people who are broadcasting negativity.

For thousands of years, a few enlightened masters at a time have balanced the negativity of the rest of humanity in this very way, since high vibration is thousands of times more powerful than low vibration. Now you can help.

Remember, the more like entertainment and the less like work it feels, the more powerful it is. If you get all serious or sad or angry about it, you're not contributing. Do it lightly and joyfully, and don't try to *make* anything happen. Try two more minutes of daydreaming right now, and make it fun!

Empty and Meaningless

ONE MORNING I woke up and noted matter-of-factly that everything seemed pointless. Since I had been in a state of pretty constant happiness with frequent blasts of bliss this was "interesting," but in my typical equanimity, I knew there was nothing wrong—I'd just witness and be with it. I went efficiently about my work and life as if nothing was different.

That's one thing that has been radically different since I began Divine Openings: nothing stops me, and I go on with what needs to be done no matter how I feel. It's as if The Presence just moves my body. Life perks along on a kind of super-efficient Divine autopilot—an invisible motor always runs.

Someone sent me a greeting card after a retreat. On it the Dalai Lama is opening a birthday present from another monk, and as he peers into the empty box, he exclaims, "Wow, just what I always wanted—NOTHING!" Pure nothing, silence, stillness is the essence of The Presence. All else is transitory form—mere stuff. The universes were birthed from No-thing into thing-ness! No-thing is fresh and freeing, a powerful state of all potentiality where you are poised in an empty gap, yet on the brink of infinite possibilities. In the retreats I take people to this fertile void of all potential during a final initiation, and new lives are born.

We hold onto "things," and define our lives by the physical world. At some stage Divine Openings graces us with the experience of No-thing-ness, and by contrast we notice how much we defined ourselves by all that stuff. As a friend packed up his possessions to move, he had to sort through and discard most of twenty years' worth of stuff. He sat on the floor, in a big pile of history, shoulders drooping. I asked him if he even wanted the stuff, and he said, "No, but it still feels like a loss to let it go." I sat quietly with him and offered, "Let that feeling be. It'll move with no resistance." "Losing" anything, particularly letting go of what defined your reality, can feel disorienting to the body and mind at first, but what you gain is space for a more expansive new reality. As much as you have wanted your life to transform, when it does it can feel joyful . . . disconcertingly unfamiliar… joyful… confusing… empty… joyful…

Meditate to experience No-thing rather than something.

Notice where emptiness is on the Instrument Panel—it's above the Tipping Point. The only reason people don't love emptiness is that it's so darn unfamiliar, and the mind resists stillness. Since I didn't resist it, I flowed through this empty and meaningless phase in about half a day! Things move through you fast when you can be with whatever is.

One day soon after, a friend hit the same stage. He said he sat staring blankly at the wall for hours, and had become quiet—very odd for him! Being an action person, he normally would have either talked about it, worked out, or found something to distract himself. For some time he had resisted giving up the fight that was so deeply ingrained in him. In his despair and fatigue, he gave up, a crack of least resistance appeared, and Grace took over and stopped him cold.

He was detached and had little to say except, "Everything feels empty and meaningless. The worst thing is nothing even seems funny. My writing depends on humor!" He grimaced. I did catch him off guard and made him laugh by saying "Hey, what an opportunity! You could go have some empty and meaningless sex!" Then I left him alone to resume his bewildered staring at the wall, to experience this auspicious death of the old, an opening to the new. He was soon on fire with more energy than ever, and on to a new phase of his business.

Our small self doesn't know what the heck is going on—great things are happening and it is not in control of them. It can get frightened! When you experience far more bliss than you're used to, even that can be disconcerting. "What if it doesn't last?" Someone shared that the acceptance she received to her music since her first Divine Opening was "almost scary." Her body was "opening up," and she had to "try to not be afraid, listen and follow." Isn't it interesting that the small-self fears the new and wonderful, even when it's what we've always wanted?

My personal experience has covered the spectrum of emotions, and I've fully experienced them all. The joy and laughter outweighed the speed bumps, and seeing things about myself I didn't like. At times it felt like a tornado had swept through and cleanly wiped the slate.

"Hmm, I don't think I'm in Kansas anymore," I murmured to myself. "So, where am I? Standing on a new and unfamiliar frontier. Oh, My God—that means no road map! No map? Heck, there are no *roads!*" I felt very powerful, but always just felt my way along.

If you want to create something new and fresh, would you paint over a canvas that was layered with thick, old paint? Or would you start on a fresh, smooth, clean, primed canvas? When you want to create something truly fresh rather than just rearranging the old ingredients, a clean, blank mind is a blessing. When you don't resist, but allow this No-mind, you are completely out of the way, and oh, Grace can lift you!

Savor and appreciate the delicious emptiness. It won't last. Let go of your busy mind and old goal-oriented way of thinking and relax for a bit. It's okay. (Everything is okay.) Inspiration does come, and then you move. Over the years I've had a number of these auspicious initiations of profound emptiness, and after each one I was soon filled with energy and inspiration to write a fresh, new, next-level book or online course, and in the retreats could lead people even higher.

What a blessing to stand empty and free in the void,
poised to create at a new level.

There is no set destiny, although you may have incarnated with some general ideas of what you wanted to experience and what your talents would be. You get to create new life and new worlds. It's your blank canvas to paint however you please. God doesn't even dictate how God will interact with you—you get to co-create that, too! Six months after my twenty-one days of silence, I once again "upgraded" my concept of God, throwing out yet another pile of concepts I realized I had picked up that were not authentic to me or had outlived their value.

After experiencing some physical pain and seeing that it was resistance (it always is), I asked within, while sitting in contemplation, "What is a truer concept of God for me *now*?" Instantly, an image of me leafing through a blank book filled with handmade paper appeared in my mind. I laughed. God is a blank book. That initiated a deeper understanding that the most pure experience of The Presence is formless. I threw out even more second-hand images and concepts and opened wider. From deep within emerged a Presence that was virtually impossible to describe. I heard the wind outside, and it seemed to be its/our breath. How we experience The Presence evolves as we evolve. Take your sweet time.

The Dark Night of the Soul

IN MY MANY YEARS of Divine Openings, some of my biggest expansions were ushered in by a dark night of the soul. It's different from the more neutral empty and meaningless, and may feel like depression or unidentifiable despair, which you can imagine is a bit surprising. At first I'll think, "I've really lost it! Something's wrong!" But when I remember to experience it with no resistance it can move very fast. Every single time, the contrast brings a new phase. It's telling me, "It's time to expand or let go yet again!" It's supposed to feel bad to hold yourself back or deny yourself expansion! One night I went to bed after a day of darkness of the soul, and a light being came in the night (it wasn't a dream) and offered a hand to lift me up.

Then came some very soothing dreams. I woke incredibly happy the next morning. Later in the day, a blind spot in my life became visible and it just cleared up with witnessing. Bliss erupted. That's typical. The dark night that classically lasted months or years was happening in mere hours for me and my clients.

A dark night of the soul is a deep, auspicious, and blessed event that takes you higher in the end. Don't panic. You haven't "lost it." You'll come through just fine. If it goes on too long and you do need Divine Openings resources, see the back of the book.

Looking Forward

JOY AND BLISS ARE NOT a product of anything; they are innate qualities of your Large Self. They can spill out of you like a fountain when you least expect it, in situations others might find miserable—like when my truck broke down. Without the interference of the mind, there is joy in anything. It's all experience. Joy isn't dependent on outer circumstances, finances, approval, love, or events; *it just is*.

Your Large Self sits in the eye of the hurricane, at peace no matter what is going on, while your small, separated self could be unhappy or in pain if things are not going right, tossed about by the winds of its own self-created storms. The small self requires things to go a certain way to be happy while your Large Self can find happiness in any situation. The small self can experience pleasure when things are going its way, but not true joy.

Once awakened, you still experience aversion to some things and attraction to others, and like some people better than others, but there is less charge and judgment (sticky glue) on it. There are simple preferences and choices. We came here to pick and choose from options and contrasts.

Emotions and phases come and go, but there is less charge on them, less resistance to them, so they don't stick; they move fluidly through you, and you don't turn pain into suffering. At first, you move in and out of blissful states, but as you stabilize, you experience the higher, finer vibrations more of the time. One minute you may feel anger or powerlessness, but you're rubberized and you quickly bounce back

The mind and body might still be concerned with survival, which is part of your basic instinct to keep you alive—but at some point you're able to de-clutch from it. You ignore it or you soothe it. You realize:

I don't have to believe everything I think.
My thoughts are not Me.
My mind and emotions are not Me.
I am not this body.

Thoughts that are not even yours may drift in from others or from Ancient Mind. If a painful thought or feeling that doesn't make any sense arises, I ask, "Is this mine?" If it's not, I offer it to The Presence, because it's too big for me, and it evaporates. If you are over-empathic and get a bad feeling that doesn't make any sense, ask, "Is this mine?" If it's not yours give it to The Presence. Each time someone does that, Ancient Mind weakens.

Your brain still works once you let go to your Divine Self; in fact, far more of it turns on and lights up, but the parts of it that become dominant are the parts that run enlightened thought. The reptilian brain at the base of the skull is soothed and less active, less dominant. The chatty parietal lobes at the sides of the skull are quieter. The more evolved frontal lobes light up and become more active, as they tune in to God-energy and produce more inspired thought.

An enormous amount of energy is used by mind-chatter. After retreats people marvel at how energized they feel after that complete break from talk and mental chatter. Your brain still works for you when you need it, but sits quiet and idle when you don't. The thoughts that do come through it are of a higher quality and more often inspired. If your mind gets busy with productive thought, that's okay. You came here to engage in this world, not sit on a cloud, empty-headed *all* of the time.

Your mind is more of a receptor for Divine Intelligence and Grace, serving you rather than running you. You keep it in a more empty, free-space state rather than storing up so many events, feelings, patterns, strategies and facts; what you need comes to you in the moment.

As you've heard, the "brain as a storage cabinet" is an outmoded notion. In the past we thought we needed to store up experiences and create patterns of response and defense so we could use them as guidance and protection in the future, but past experience is obviously not the best guide if we want to go beyond the past. Direct knowing is available in the moment we need it. Too often, past experience limits what is possible. Now we're free of the past, and human consciousness is expanding daily.

Enlightenment may or may not bring on mystical gifts like psychic ability, channeling, healing, and mystical visions. The unique gifts that do unfold will be perfect for you.

You don't need flashy phenomena to be fully awakened. If your heart opens and you become quietly loving and compassionate to your entire family, this is more valuable than clairvoyance or visions, and does as much good for the world.

My experiences have been perfect for me, and I am fully satisfied with them. Speeding through life seeking wild experiences is pointless. I am here!

Measure your wealth in enlightenment, happiness, and love.

You're Never "Finished"

CAN YOU IMAGINE God complaining, "Geez, when will this creation ever be done? I have worked and worked and worked on it for eons, and still it's not done! When am I ever going to be able to relax and retire?" Sounds silly, doesn't it? But that's what we do. We want it to be done, finished, perfect, over. For what? What else do we have to do with eternity? Enjoy NOW.

Creation expands forever; the game is verdant, rich, multi-faceted, infinite creation. The Creator in us cannot stop creating. Energy moves through us, generating expansion, creating an exhilarating current that our Large Self rides for fun. When we learn to ride it for fun too, we've mastered the game. When we march through life trying to get somewhere, there is no joy, and we are out of alignment with our Large Self.

Sometimes people who are progressing more slowly ask me why others they read about on our website have such miraculous results so quickly. The people who get free and happy the fastest:

- Let go of everything they knew from the past.

- Stop seeking and processing, and don't dilute Divine Openings with other things.

- Enjoy life.

- Appreciate and soften around all feelings.

- Take everything within to The Presence instead of talking about it to other people, whether friends or therapists. Stop trying to get someone else to make it go away or fix it for you.

- Stop telling their old stories. Period.

- Claim responsibility for their own reality, even when they don't yet understand how they created a particular thing. They say, "I created it," in a kind, compassionate way.

- They don't try to figure it out intellectually.

- Make a powerful decision to stop looking to the outer world for validation or clarity.

- Commit without reservation to create their own reality, and stick to that.

- Don't take score too soon. Focus only on what's working, not what isn't. Delete "failures" and don't count them.

- Practice appreciation and raving daily.

- Minimize complaining and wrong-making.

- Read this book again, letting in more as your consciousness expands.

- Prioritize happiness.

- Set a strong intention to slow down and savor life rather than speeding through it.

- Keep happily moving through the Divine Openings Online Portals of Awakening rather than stagnating or settling.

Note that none of this involves working on yourself!

Most people move quickly with Divine Openings, and some take longer. One student who described herself as resistant realized after over two years of Divine Openings that she'd been trying every trick to not have to feel deeply. Her fearful small self thought there must be some loophole, some way around it. She didn't have childhood trauma, she was simply running from messy human feelings; a perfectionist wanting life to be perfect. She began to open up, let go, and live life, but still hadn't ventured into relationship—she was procrastinating about dating, thinking she'd have to kiss too many toads.

Three years into Divine Openings she sent me a little gift with a note saying she was embarking on a new career, and that a man in her apartment complex knocked on her door one day and asked her out, and they've been together since. It happened just that easily, sans frog kissing, and they are happy.

Another student complained that her sister had gotten the full bliss of Divine Openings but she wasn't getting it. She persistently held onto the story that all her problems were her husband's fault, and it was quite comical watching this tiny irritated woman bossing her big burly, easy-going guy around at the retreat, but he was infinitely patient. Finally after two years, she gleefully wrote me that she claimed responsibility for her own happiness, and she and her husband were in love like teenagers again, their relationship better than it had been in twenty years. Yes, and she finally got "the bliss."

When you stop waiting for someone else to change, stop seeking some magic bullet that will save you from ever feeling bad again, and start living life now, you can expand forever with ease and joy. However long your awakening takes is okay when you know your enjoyment of each moment of eternity is all that matters. You know there is no goal except to be alive and awake right now.

Make peace now with your ever-expanding, never-ending journey through eternity. Laugh at the old notion of ever getting somewhere, becoming perfect, or "getting it all done." You'll die with an undone to-do list, but since there is no death, it doesn't matter. You, infinite being, are never done.

Once awakened, many people visit our website like a favorite hangout. Wanting ongoing inspiration and compatible energy is natural—I need it too. So much of the input we get from the world isn't uplifting and doesn't support this awakened life we've chosen to live. We've created our own lit up and supportive "world" at www.DivineOpenings.com, and DivineOpenings.de for Germany, Austria, and Switzerland.

Do share with those you love before you forget how you got free! Share the book and website with them so they have all of the same support and advantages you had.

Divine Opening

THIS IS SOUL'S DANCE, the essence of doing your soul's dance full out.
Gaze at this image for one minute, then close your eyes
and savor for fifteen or more minutes.

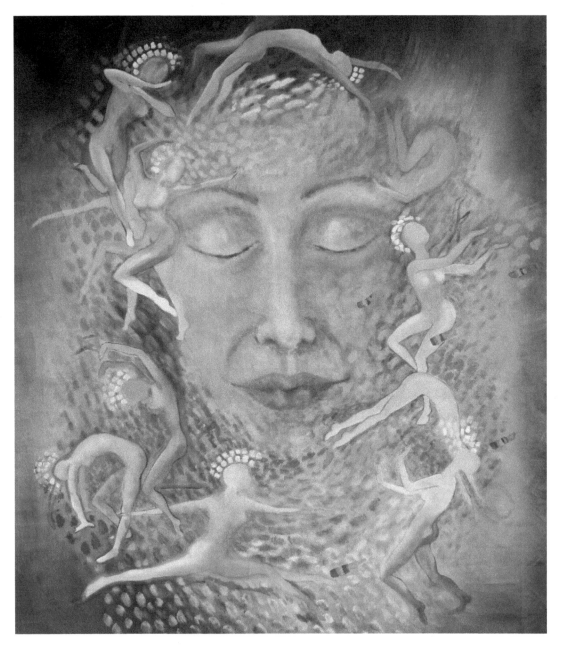

Figure 10—Soul's Dance, painting by Lola Jones

How The Unfolding Might Go For You

YOU WILL BEGIN to glimpse a new dimension of living within weeks with Divine Openings, if you're doing the activities and not just reading; if you're feeling, going within, staying focused, and not diluting it. Some people take longer. This book, which is at Level One, usually gets people out of suffering, anxiety, and worry, and it gets most people to quiet joy and inner peace or higher. Now you have a whole new awareness of how you're creating your reality, but most importantly, you know how to raise your vibration and feel better. That allows you to increasingly manifest more deliberately.

A single Divine Opening may have a delayed effect of days or even months depending on what it needs to do within you. For example, you might read the whole book and not feel much at all. Then days, weeks, or months later the Grace has melted through mountains of invisible resistance, and you have a huge awakening, seemingly out of the blue. If you'd wandered back to seeking, you might attribute it to the wrong thing, then it gets really confusing. Seeking and working on yourself reverses the awakening, by definition. You can't be awakened and seeking at the same time. It's like being both lost and found—you can't be both.

This initiation to enlightenment is just a beginning. When you wake up in the morning, you still have sleep in your eyes and you still may not see clearly. So it is with your spiritual awakening. You get the bliss of enlightenment; then you gradually learn to bring it down to earth, to your relationships, your work, your play, your whole life. A process of refinement of your human self occurs.

Enlightenment can happen in a flash, but the retraining and refinement of your mind can take time. Once you're stabilized, you will be like a mighty oak, a solid support for others. But until then, tend that tender new green shoot with care, giving yourself support and inspiration, nourishment and upliftment.

I invite you to read this book again slowly once you finish it. During the second reading, one man realized he'd thought it was too good to be true, so his belief that it couldn't be true held him back, and that's why he wasn't seeing physical changes in his life yet. The second time he let go of his doubts to give it a real chance, felt deeply into it, did the activities, and his life transformed. Some resist doing the activities the first time but do them on a later reading once Grace has softened and worked on them in the meantime.

In my experience with many thousands of people, they rise, stabilize, and maintain their awakening best if they read this book a couple of times and then move on to the next levels. It can be hard for the mind to imagine there could actually be more, but there is always more, so don't just settle for a bit of progress.

Your "pipes" expand gradually, and at each level you can let more Grace in. As your consciousness expands you can hear and see things at each level that you were not ready for before. You'll feel, let go of, and do things you resisted before. Your conscious mind has benefited from this step by step retraining, and time to see the positive proof of it.

Life is a delicious eternal unfolding—savor and appreciate every single step.

Stay Immersed

LIFE WILL OFFER TO IMMERSE YOU in all kinds of useless and even destructive things. Choose carefully what to immerse yourself in! Play with these practices daily with a light attitude and get any support you need until you feel pretty consistently stable, and eventually astonishingly great. Then do maintenance practices in a fun, playful way. Stay off that healing-seeking-and-working-on-yourself-hamster-wheel!

The *Thirty Ways To Raise Your Altitude* page near the end of this book serves as a quick guide to staying high and continuing to expand. There's a Daily Pleasure Practice page, too. Create your own unique Pleasure Practice routine and refresh it as needed to keep it fun and alive. Keep playing with it until you've formed solid new habits. Pleasure Practices are just a part of how I live now. My mind is sharp and efficient, even at 64 as of the 2018 edition. I feel fabulous and love my physical workouts. My creativity and energy is flowing.

Since Divine Openings, I'm on the automatic upgrade program. Challenges come and go quickly. I don't get stuck for long. We become more self-correcting, self-healing, and self-guided as we go, but if you need help with a blind spot, big challenge, or area of resistance, help is here. Some of you will need more social support. I get massages because they feel good and help my body flow this constantly increasing energy. A chiropractor, acupuncturist, naturopath, and some Divine Openings Guides supported me on a couple of physical things.

You may see progress in certain areas faster than others. Perhaps you become liberated first in your relationships, then money, but last in your physical health. The ideal relationship came last for me. It comes when it comes. Complaining that it's not here yet sends you backward, away from it. Appreciate, enjoy, let go! If you relax your grip, let go to the flow, and are having a great time, *you're there now!*

Stick to it. I've watched some people have some astounding experiences with Divine Openings, get really high and free, then wander off into seeking and get lost again. Someone said to me after wandering off and then coming back to Divine Openings, "Well, I thought if Divine Openings is this good, adding a ton of other spiritual energies would be even better. It wasn't."

I've also said it this way: if you just met your ideal mate, would you keep dating other people for years?

If you rely on others to fix, clear, make you feel better, connect you to The Presence, or heal your emotions instead of using your Instrument Panel, you remain dependent and outer focused. Divine Openings will *always* point you back inside to your Large Self.

Once you're sure you won't give any power away, you can let in care and contribution from various people in your life. An occasional reading with a *gifted, high vibration* psychic can even help, but be careful what you take in; they're only human. Remember, *they're only reading what you're creating* with the vibration you are radiating right now. Change your vibration, change the future.

One thing will surely happen, and it may shock you as well as delight you: as you open and awaken further, many of your old desires will simply dissolve. So many of those desires came from your small self or societal conditioning, and now it's clear you never really needed them, and they wouldn't have made you happy anyway. Deep peace and causeless bliss more than replaces those illusory things. After a year or so, look back at what you wrote in front of the book.

Most of all, relax, get a real life, not the life everyone else says is best, and enjoy it. Life is for living, not "seeking so that *someday* you can begin to live." *You can live now.*

Support and Further Expansion

WHEN I LED CORPORATE TRAININGS, I studied "learning theory" so I could be more effective with all types of learning styles. It was particularly important when companies like IBM sent me in to train the toughest of all audiences: super smart high-tech people who weren't one bit excited about learning people skills! To keep their attention and get them to buy into and retain the material, I had to learn how to engage all learning styles and employ all learning channels: visual, auditory, kinesthetic (feeling,) and sensory.

Those fifteen years taught me that most people learn faster and retain it longer when they see it, hear it, have it demonstrated, and then *participate* in active application of it *rather than just reading it*. This explains the wild popularity of YouTube, Facebook, the Internet, TV, and the decline in radio and reading books. It explains why reading even the best spiritual and self-help books works for some and not at all for others.

I am blessed that Grace makes this more than just a book—an experience—but there is still more to Divine Openings than can be conveyed in a book.

If everyone could learn and grow dramatically by written materials alone, IBM wouldn't pay millions each year to trainers; they'd just have their employees read books. Kids wouldn't go to school; they'd just stay home and read assignments. No, we know that experiential, guided, entertaining, multi-media learning is far more effective, goes deeper, and is retained better.

Learning theory explains why people clamored for an audio version of this book, and why I happily recorded it in my own voice, and had a Guide record the German version. We got so blissed out doing it!

Most people feel the energy more intensely when they hear my voice, or see me teach and counsel in audios and videos. The eye contact with me is powerful. It's as if The Presence is looking at you. The most intense energy of all is from total immersion with me in retreats.

I've spent twelve years lovingly creating an enormous multi-media website with audios and videos to actively guide you through all this book's groundbreaking tools and methods and the hundreds more I've developed since then through my own endless evolution and expansion.

Countless people have told us they didn't want this book to end, and were happy Divine Openings offered continuity after it. Transforming people's lives is my life's passion and commitment. I offer everything I have, knowing fully what it can do, and with no attachment to who lets it all in or not.

Some people are content after a few readings of this book to simply be out of suffering and struggle —feeling good for the first time in their lives—they don't want to reach for more. Or they still hold limits on how much more is possible *for them*; their pipes and their beliefs aren't yet stretched to allow more. But if you wish, the complete Divine Openings works are available to you on our website for support, structure, and interactivity.

If you wish to express your appreciation, and help others find this book,
please post a review at Amazon.com or Amazon.de.
Readers' generosity in sharing DivineOpenings.com or .de and this book
has changed thousands of lives all over the world.

Epilogue

I'VE UPDATED *Things Are Going Great In My Absence* many times, because Divine Openings, like life, constantly expands and evolves me. While I can never include all the constant new updates in the books, the Online Course Portals are always full of up to the minute material. Divine Openings will apparently never stop evolving—it's a living thing. In my wildest dreams I never imagined I would create more than twenty-one Online Course Portals, but the fresh new downloads keep coming in response to people asking for more. They don't want the adventure, the support and connection to end.

My very being is designed to make fresh, new Energy/Light/Intelligence accessible to this planet, so for the Tenth Anniversary of this now classic book, I updated it yet again, then again! Most of the unstoppable flow of entirely new leading-edge material and new energy downloads go into the online courses because a website is easily changeable, and again, because most people absorb it more deeply through a live voice and pictures. There's a wealth of free material, audios, videos, blogs and more than fifty free articles on the site.

Many lovingly call the website "The Mothership" because it's an enormous "world" that supports us in this chosen reality we enjoy so much. They visit to enjoy, immerse themselves, to uplift others, be inspired, and participate. We've all made many deep and lasting friendships on the member Forum, in courses, and most deeply, in retreats.

I've talked about how we can create worlds. Well, DivineOpenings.com and .de is a virtual world so huge it practically exerts its own gravitational pull, as evidenced by the number of people who first found the site when it just popped up on their screen, when they weren't touching the computer or searching! I know—it amazes me too. Many people make it their home page and start their day exploring and soaking up the high resonance that's now their "home frequency." It's a place where you're understood and can feel at home.

When *Things Are Going Great In My Absence* was first written, people said they'd never seen anything like it—it was unique and revolutionary. Now many famous authors, healers, and teachers have adopted some of it in their own work—you'll see pieces of it out there. Yet Divine Openings is most powerful in its pure, *complete*, unadulterated, undiluted form. The concepts are only 10% of it—Grace does 90%. In this book and at DivineOpenings.com and DivineOpenings.de it's presented in its purest, most potent form.

People in over 150 countries were introduced to Divine Openings as people generously shared their experiences. When it was translated to German in 2012 , the German speaking world lovingly embraced Divine Openings, and they bring me over twice a year to lead retreats.

When I began taking singing lessons in 2009 it was all for fun. Now I've created fifteen uplifting original songs Tom Hopkins and others, and I'm co-creating new ecstatic chants for you now. The inspiration to paint Divine Art comes and goes.

Confessions Of A Cowgirl Guru, a laugh-out-loud humor book, flowed out of me because I love to laugh and make others laugh. I still dream of making a film about Divine Openings. I'll keep merrily expanding and evolving (but not working on myself ever again) till the day I happily depart the planet.

With Endless Love, Ease, and Grace,

Lola

PS – Near the end of 2017, after this most recent book update was handed to the printer, I was once again blessed with fresh, new inspiration. The Five Portals of Awakening were born—a step-by-step guided journey that gives you the Keys to Awakening, which you then use to pass through each Portal of Awakening, all the way to spiritual maturity.

It cannot be adequately described in words, it is best experienced in the new videos now being added to the Five Portals of Awakening Online Courses (formerly called the Levels 1 through 5 Online Courses.)

Support for Ongoing Evolution

This book is part of Portal 1, the Foundation. It is completed by the leading-edge Portal 1 Online Course, which guides you through the First of Awakening. This beautiful step by step path is outlined on DivineOpenings.com, or in German at DivineOpenings.de.

5 Day Silent Retreats: In California and Europe. Five days in Lola's powerful field of resonance is the most profound experience of Divine Openings. Issues melt away by Grace. See Live Retreats at DivineOpenings.com or .de

Subscribe to our newsletter at DivineOpenings.com/aweber to receive fresh energy, inspirational articles, gifts, updates, and news of retreats and events. We never, ever share your data. Thank you.

Things Are Going Great Audio Book, 13 hours of enjoyment and live energy, read by Lola in English and by a Divine Openings student in German. See Books at DivineOpenings.com or .de.

Book 2: *Living Large: Mastering Your Power of Intention* (formerly titled Watch Where You Point That Thing) It is completed by Portal 2 Online. In English and German.

Divine Openings Online Study:
Portal 1 Online Course, offered in English and German. Our online multi-media courses provide powerful immersion, support, fresh energy, conscious mind training, and entertainment for the mind to support your upward progress. As the mind always wants more, they help prevent falling back into addictive seeking or modality mixing.

Portal 2 Online Course, in English and German. Master your power of intention with ease and Grace, and soar higher into a life of fun and fulfilment.

Portal 3 Online-21 Days of Deepening; Portal 4-Jumping the Matrix; and Portal 5-Mastery Online complete the Five Portals of Awakening. These are in English only as of 2018, but courses are steadily being translated to German.

Diving In Audio/Video Set —A foundational Divine Openings tool, in English and German. The twenty-plus audios and videos gently walk you through the processes. It's easier to let go when you don't have to think at the same time. Lola's and other Guides' voices invoke a powerful vortex that soothes and softens resistance until you can Dive In successfully on your own. See Talk Audios in the site menu.

Live Interactive Webinar Series with Lola, see Webinars in the site menu.

Divine Openings Guide Certification, for those who want to give and teach Divine Openings, and is also popular for those who just want advanced coaching. In English and German.

Private Sessions. Certified Guides zero in on precisely what you need. See Sessions on the site.

Enlightened Business Online Course, in English and German. Get more prosperous!

The Art of Love and Sex: Tantra, in English and German. If deep, loving, spiritual sex is not part of your path, what are you waiting for?

Check "What's New?" on the website often for new audios, videos, courses, articles, blogs, features, quotes, and events.

Lola's Original Music. The Presence moves through Lola to create inspired music in many genres, dance, pop, blues, to spiritual. Download them with ease.

Lola's Art: See Art in the menu. If you wish to brighten the energy in your space, the Divine Art is available in 8x10 high-resolution prints, large poster-size reproductions, and prints on canvas. Commissioned Paintings with Divine Energy can be channeled for you if Lola has time and inspiration. admin@lolajones.com, support@DivineOpeningsGermany.com

More Enlightening Books from Lola Jones

Living Large: Mastering Your Power of Intention. Formerly titled Watch Where You Point That Thing. In German it's titled: *Du bist so viel größer als du denkst! Anleitung zum Erschaffen eines wundervollen Lebens.*

Confessions Of A Cowgirl Guru—A humor collection inspired by Lola's life, loves, and observations about the holistic culture and the metaphysical life.

Divine Openings Quotes—A beautiful book of wisdom; heart-opening, funny, surprising.

Dating To Change Your Life — This book is pre-Divine Openings, but it's good… and it's funny. Makes dating fun, transforming your life in the process. Get happy and find your partner faster.

Coming: a new as yet untitled book that condenses the essence of Mastery into concise words and images.

50+ free articles: www.DivineOpenings.com/spiritual-awakening-articles
If a page is available in German, there'll always be a <u>Deutsch</u> link at top of the web page
Or click Free in the menu. Scroll down to 50+ free articles.

Special free bonus support pages:
www.DivineOpenings.com/divine-mother-hug
www.DivineOpenings.com/spiritual-enlightenment-processes

Contact: admin@LolaJones.com, support@DivineOpeningsGermany.com
Send raves and reviews: celebrate@lolajones.com

Thirty Ways To Raise Your Altitude

Notice that these all feel good and *none of them are work!* Do them for joy, and not just to solve problems. They help you retrain yourself to operate at a higher frequency. There is no limit to how high you can go and how good you can feel. Use them as part of your Daily Pleasure Practice. Some of these methods will work starting from anywhere on the Altimeter. Others will work best when you are already flying fairly high. Try different ones until one works.

1. **Breathe for pleasure:** Sit or lie down. Put a tiny smile on your lips. Arch your back slightly as you inhale for five counts, and bend your spine gently forward as you breathe out for five counts. Silently say "yessss" on the inhale and breathe "ahhh" on the exhale. Breathe easy for five to fifteen minutes.

2. **Soothe yourself:** Move energy up step by step on a subject by telling yourself a better story about that subject. Be soft on yourself. "Where I am is where I am. I can get anywhere from wherever I am. This is temporary. Everything changes. Things always work out."

3. **Date With The Divine:** Silence. Tech detox: no television, telephone, computer or email. The ultimate date with The Divine is the 5 Day Silent Bliss Retreat.

4. **Fork in the road:** Choose the better-feeling thought or action and feel the immediate relief.

5. **Turn your body:** Get up and turn your whole body in a different direction. Turn away from what you don't want, toward what you *do* want, and feel the difference in your body.

6. **Choose your focus:** In every moment, choose only past, present, or future thoughts that feel good when you think about them.

7. **Move your body:** Act out each emotion on the Instrument Panel to get your energy moving in a dynamic way, and get you out of your head. Download Lola's original music at www.DivineOpenings.com

8. **Daydream:** For entertainment only! This is not work. What you want is already "given," created, and done. Your job is to vibrate, think, and feel in harmony with it so it can materialize.

9. **Add humor:** Cultivate humor and fun friends. Read, watch, and seek out more humor.

10. **Rave about it!** Think of everything there is to appreciate about a person or subject, yourself or your life in general, and rave on and on about it. Do this out loud or silently.

11. **Dive In:** Drop the story about it. Say "yes" to the unwanted feeling as you breathe allowing and acceptance into it. Any feeling fully felt rises.

12. **Prostrate:** Lay it down at the feet of The Presence. Breathe deeply through it for pleasure until you feel a lift.

13. **Dream Intention:** Make a list of everything you want, put it to dream assignment to get yourself out of the way. Sleep easy, knowing it's being handled. Follow what feels good the next day and watch for subtle guidance in any form. Drop any timetable and don't take score. It's done.

14. **Put it on your God List:** Make a list of what you want and give the whole list over to The Presence, who already knows—putting it on the list just *helps you get out of the way!*

15. **Take a break/give it a rest!** Take your focus completely off the specific or difficult subject and do something that already feels good. This gets you out of the way and raises your general vibration.

16. **Vacation:** Take a vacation or a mini-vacation and let go of "work." No phones, no computers, no effort. Break your routine entirely and relax.

17. **Pet pampering:** Play with your pets. Get in tune with how joyful they are.

18. **Witness:** Witness your body, then your thoughts, then your emotions. No judging, no fixing.

19. **Ask your Large Self:** "What do you know and feel about this?" "What would work better?" "How could I experience this differently?" "What amazing development is next for me?"

20. **Chat casually with your Large Self often:** "Look at that… What do you think?... I'm thinking this… I appreciate that… That was easy wasn't it?"

21. **Simply focus on your Large Self:** It never goes away—you do! Go home to it! Focus points energy and builds momentum. Let go of what should happen and just do your 10%.

22. **Take score of wins.** Focus on how far you've come and what has worked out.

23. **Don't take score if the point's not in your favor:** Delay taking score of yet-un-materialized things, or things that didn't work. Say, "Next!" or "It's still coming! My job is to raise my altitude and feel good about it."

24. **Feel good first:** Do two things that feel good to you, then do your "must do's" afterward. Luxuriate in the bed before you rise. Take a bath, walk, sing, garden, etc.

25. **Have it now:** Put yourself in the feeling of "having it now." Gather information, visit places physically and "test drive" any desire you have that feels too far away.

26. **Claim your power**: At each little elevation say, "I created just a little relief! If I can do that I can do anything! All it takes is one step like that at a time."
—When unwanted manifestations show up, say, "I created that! How powerful I am!"
—When things you do want show up, say, "I created that! How powerful I am!"

27. **Be happy now:** You think being somewhere else or having things be different will make you happy. Take the short cut and be happy now. Then Law of Attraction can give you more of it.

28. **Give up control:** Mind your own business. Let other people, the world, and things outside you be, do, and have whatever they choose. Choose your reality independent of that, knowing that no one can create in your reality or hold you back—only you can.

29. **Easy button:** Hit your "easy button" every time something goes well or comes easy! Order them online at Staples.com. Give them to friends!

30. **Meditation:** There is no resistance while you're not thinking. Any simple, easy breath meditation will take you deeper into your core essence. The Online Course Portals give you many, many meditations so you can find the ones that suit you best.

Sample Daily Pleasure Practice

Morning:
1. **Breathe-For-Pleasure:** There is no resistance while you're not thinking. Sit. Smile slightly. Minutely arch your back a bit as you inhale, and bend your spine forward a tiny bit as you exhale. In your mind, say "yes" on the inhale, and "ahhh," on the exhale. Enjoy for five to fifteen minutes.

2. **Rave about it:** Focus on appreciating yourself, everything, and everyone you can for five minutes.

3. **Daydream:** Playfully imagine how you want your day to go or how you want it to feel, just for entertainment. (Don't take score if it doesn't immediately go that way. Take score only on what did go well.) Pleasantly anticipate how you'd like each individual activity to go before you begin. Line up the energy, and action flows smoother.

4. **Pleasure Practices:** Do things that feel good—listen or move to Lola's Divine Music (found at www.DivineOpenings.com) or others, sing, garden, take a bath, take a walk, pet your cat. You'll be more productive. You can always feel even better.

As You Go About Your Day:
1. **Inspired action:** Do the actions you are inspired to do first. Act when it feels guided, when your altitude is high on that subject, unless there is an absolute deadline like bills or taxes.

2. **Take meditation breaks:** Sit quietly and be aware of the gaps between each breath. Or the way the breath arcs between each inhale and exhale, as if in a circle. Especially when it seems you must rush or work harder: Stop. Tune inward and get in alignment with your Large Self before taking action.

Evening:
1. **Pleasure Practices:** Do something that feels good to you, that you will feel good about long term.

2. **Move your body and play:** Dance, walk, sing, run with the dog, bike, or swim. Wiggle, jump, laugh, be goofy. Moving the body in dynamic and unusual ways unsticks the mind. Get out of your head.

3. **Savor:** Luxuriate in smells, sights, sensations, touch, and sounds. Enjoy sensual moments wherever you find or create them.

Before bed:
1. **Rave:** Focus on appreciating yourself, everything, and everyone you can for five minutes.

2. **Witnessing Meditation:** Be mindful of your body, then your thoughts, then your emotions. Just sit and watch the sensations float by with no judgment or attachment.

3. **Set Dream Intentions.** Relax, tiny smile, snuggle in, and let go.

Add your own favorites. Update it often so it stays fresh.

More comments from readers. Thousands more reviews on the website are offered to give you hope that it can indeed happen for you. See Reviews in the menu:

When I first started Divine Openings nine years ago, I was in despair. I must have listened to each of Lola's recorded audio sessions five times over... they soothed me, I learned from them, and they helped me lift my vibration out of despair and on to a steady climb. Those recordings were invaluable, and I'm so, so thankful that I had them to help me navigate! These days I live in bliss, my family is awesome, and my work is a joy as well as extremely successful and profitable. Donna Wetterstrand, Canada

Awareness of how I've been resistant to receiving came up strongly. I asked God to soften me and then that 'download' happened again immediately, and He held me and showed me exactly what to do. I've never experienced automatic writing before—what an awesome experience. Thank you for helping me remember my way home as I'd gotten lost lately. —Blessings to you, Michelle Wolff

So much has happened so fast that I can barely even articulate it. I am just so grateful that I found your work on the net. Why, why, why doesn't Oprah know about you? Your work is the obvious next step to the Tolle stuff because of its practical, down to earth, how-to accessibility. I can just imagine a Divine Opening on the Oprah show! I'm sending you love. —Donna Wetterstrand, Canada

I just listened to your trauma and abuse audio on the Diving In series, and it is one of the most exquisite pieces of therapy I've ever heard. I've been in this field for these many years and nothing I have seen, heard, done, or delivered myself even comes close. Another WOW! —Donna

The energy was incredible. I had to go slower than one opening every two weeks—I found myself moving very quickly. I would look back at things I did just a week or two ago and say to myself, why did I handle it that way when I know it could have been handled like this…. then I realized that a week or two ago I wasn't in the place I am now! I feel less stressed, more like I am floating through life— not all the time, but more and more. Thank you! —Eleanor

As you gave the Divine Opening (on the phone) I was aware of my feet . . . and I saw in my mind's eye, the hands of Jesus washing them. The sensation of a breeze softly blowing around my ankles and feet started and continues even now, seven hours later. Sweet! —Julie, Arizona

I've had some significant movement. I love your unshakable faith, your playfulness, that you are a 'powerhouse renegade,' and how your wisdom cuts through to profound truth. —Much Love, Naraya

Lola, everything I want . . . It's not coming . . . It's already HERE! I just have to KEEP letting it in! IT feels so amazing. —Love, Nicole

Many times I felt like people who I love were inside me and I could feel their love for me, also. —Ana

My body is changing from within. Sometimes I can't eat foods I used to like, and I don't want those foods. So I am losing a bit of weight now too. —Edith

Thanks for keeping up with me, as I probably need supervision (just kidding.) Well, after much groundwork and trial and error, everything is falling into place for my business. I'm retired, but like all intense people, retirement means just having enough free time to start another business. I've searched for a teacher of my kind of spirituality. I know this is "it." Nothing else has ever felt this way for me. —All my love and gratitude, Kathy

I gave the book to my mom in Georgia who is 78. She called me yesterday all excited about her first Divine Opening. What she explained to me was that she felt a pulse run through her whole body, even in her fingertips. Then she saw a light around a black hole, she explained that things were going into the black hole really fast, and then it closed up and disappeared. It is going to be fun to keep sharing these experiences with my Mom. I am giving a book to my daughter Rachel, 24. You will be touching the lives of 3 generations in my family. —Carey Waters

My husband and I have a code word—"the Book"—we say it when one of us is crabby or aggravated. Then we smile and laugh a little because we both know what it means. Sincerely and with love, —Julie